Contents

List of contributors

Martin Godfrey
Public Relations, UK

Charlotte Green
Newsreader
BBC Radio 4
London, UK

Angela Hall
Emeritus Reader in Clinical Communication
St George's
University of London
London, UK

George M. Hall
Professor of Anaesthesia
St George's
University of London
London, UK

William Harrop-Griffiths
Consultant Anaesthetist
Imperial College Healthcare NHS Trust
London, UK

Roger Horton
Emeritus Professor of Neuropharmacology
St George's
University of London
London, UK

Sir Alexander Macara
Public Health Physician
Bristol, UK

Alan Maryon-Davis
Honorary Professor of Public Health
King's College London
London, UK

Peter McCrorie
Professor of Medical Education
St George's
University of London
London, UK

Mal Morgan
Emeritus Reader in Anaesthetic Practice
Imperial College London
London, UK

Philip M. Sedgwick
Senior Lecturer in Medical Statistics
St George's
University of London
London, UK

Richard Smith
Executive Director, UnitedHealth Europe
London, UK

Sir Terry Wogan
Broadcaster
London, UK

How to Present at Meetings

THIRD EDITION

Edited by

George M. Hall
Professor of Anaesthesia
St George's, University of London
London, UK

Neville Robinson
Consultant Anaesthetist
Northwick Park and St Mark's Hospitals
Harrow, UK

WILEY-BLACKWELL
A John Wiley & Sons, Ltd., Publication

BMJ|Books

This edition first published 2012 © 2012 by George M. Hall and Neville Robinson

BMJ Books is an imprint of BMJ Publishing Group Limited, used under licence by Blackwell Publishing which was acquired by John Wiley & Sons in February 2007. Blackwell's publishing programme has been merged with Wiley's global Scientific, Technical and Medical business to form Wiley-Blackwell.

Registered Office: John Wiley & Sons, Ltd, The Atrium, Southern Gate, Chichester, West Sussex, PO19 8SQ, UK

Editorial Offices: 9600 Garsington Road, Oxford, OX4 2DQ, UK
      The Atrium, Southern Gate, Chichester, West Sussex, PO19 8SQ, UK
      111 River Street, Hoboken, NJ 07030-5774, USA

For details of our global editorial offices, for customer services and for information about how to apply for permission to reuse the copyright material in this book please see our website at www.wiley.com/wiley-blackwell

The right of the author to be identified as the author of this work has been asserted in accordance with the UK Copyright, Designs and Patents Act 1988.

Library of Congress Cataloging-in-Publication Data

How to present at meetings / [edited by] George M. Hall, Peter Neville Robinson. – 3rd ed.
    p. ; cm.
    Includes bibliographical references and index.
    ISBN 978-0-470-65458-3 (pbk.)
  1. Communication in medicine.   2. Lectures and lecturing.   3. Communication of technical information.
I. Hall, George M. (George Martin)   II. Robinson, Neville.
  [DNLM: 1. Communication.   2. Congresses as Topic.   3. Professional Competence. 4. Speech.   HF 5718.22]
  R118.H69 2012
  610.69′6–dc23

                                    2011024960

A catalogue record for this book is available from the British Library.

This book is published in the following electronic formats: ePDF 9781119962090; Wiley Online Library 9781119962120; ePub 9781119962106

Set in 9.5/12pt Minion by Aptara Inc., New Delhi, India.
Printed in Singapore by Ho Printing Singapore Pte Ltd

1   2012

How to Present
at Meetings

Preface to the third edition

We are pleased that Sir Terry Wogan has kindly agreed to write a foreword for the third edition and we are most grateful for his wit and wisdom. In this edition Philip Sedgwick has contributed a new chapter on the production and presentation of posters for scientific meetings and William Harrop-Griffiths has written a chapter that should enable all novice presenters to cope with the idiosyncrasies of PowerPoint presentations. We are most appreciative of all the other contributors who have revised their chapters and thank them for their continuing support.

G. M. Hall and Neville Robinson

Preface to the second edition

The call for a second edition of this book has enabled the authors to revise their chapters. I am delighted that Charlotte Green, a doyen amongst BBC Radio announcers and newsreaders, has contributed a chapter on how to present a talk. I have encouraged overlap between authors on the basis that repetition aids learning and understanding; a view supported by two eminent medical educationalists in Chapter 1. Once again I am grateful for the enthusiasm of the contributors; the book's success is their success.

G. M. Hall

Preface to the first edition

Many trainees in medicine, while competent in their speciality, struggle to give a good presentation at a meeting. The aim of this book is to provide a basic framework around which a proficient talk can be built. The content covers not only the essential parts of a presentation, preparation, visual aids and computer-generated slides, but also provides advice on how to sell a message, how to appear on stage and how to deal with questions. All contributors are experienced speakers and provide simple didactic advice. I am grateful for their enthusiastic cooperation.

G. M. Hall

Foreword: Wogan's wisdom: how to 'read' an audience

The first thing to remember is that Audiences Differ and Presenters Die. Accept this, the first principle of public speaking, and you can move into the Circle of Fear. Make no mistake about it, if you agree to address a meeting, you will know fear, such as you have never known before.... So, my second word of advice is: Don't do it! What so-called friend conned you into doing it in the first place? You could be at home with your feet up and a nice cup of tea, enjoying "Strictly Come Dancing", and here you are, already in a flop-sweat, with a baying crowd ready to rush the platform. That's the way I feel anyway, every time I'm foolish enough to agree to make a speech, at everything from a Rotarian gathering to a crowd of sneering conventioneers.

Mind you, there are audiences, and there are audiences. If you're addressing a Prayer meeting, there's no need for a racy gag to open proceedings. Just bring your rosary beads. If it's a Board meeting, as long as they have coffee and biscuits, all they'll want are the facts. Don't even bother smiling. If it's a Meeting of Minds, everyone will agree with every word you say anyway. But if it's a crowd, you'd better gird your loins.... I realise that you're expecting me to regale you with many a shrewdly-observed observation on how to worm your way into the hearts and minds of the numpties sitting expectantly before you, and I wish I could, but if it were that simple, the world and his wife would be at it. And you know as well as I do, having attended more than your share of gatherings, from lunches, to dinners, to bar-mitzvahs, that public speaking is an arcane art, and one bestowed on very few. I know of many comedians and presenters whose fame on TV and Radio is legendary, but who run a mile when asked to speak at a charity or celebrity lunch or dinner. For it's a completely different animal from standing on a stage, or in front of a camera, telling gags. It's much more difficult when they've had a few drinks....

A couple of years ago, I was the 'turn' at a big 'do' at the Grosvenor House Hotel, London, not known as an easy gig. It's a huge hall, the tables are all around you and even above you. You can't make eye contact with anybody, except those immediately in front of you, and they're talking to each other anyway. Still, it all went swimmingly; I played the audience like a stringed instrument and took away my brown envelope packed with crisp onecers with a light heart. There's no feeling like it, when you go down a storm. Just as there's nothing quite like dying like a dog in front of a couple of thousand disillusioned diners. Which is exactly what happened, the following year, at exactly the same 'do' in exactly the same blasted ballroom. The comedian who'd kicked things off hadn't gone well and, as ever with his ilk, couldn't let it lie, but continued to struggle well beyond his allotted hour. I came on a half an hour later than I had the previous triumphant year, the audience had had a couple of more drinks and it was Goodbye, Mr Chips. . . .

So, you see why it's not a bit of use me, or anybody else, trying to tell you how to interpret an audience's mood. There are too many imponderable factors beyond your control. They may not like the look of you, for a start. However, while you're there, here's a couple of tips that might save you from suffering too much:

- Always go on first. If you follow an eejit, it's hard to pick up the pieces, and if you're following some unknown who's played a blinder, it's even worse.
- Unless you're completely confident and relaxed, don't smile. You'll frighten the horses.
- Open with an apposite quotation, not with a gag. It makes you look intelligent.
- If you must tell a joke, keep it short. One of your famous long routines may set the boys in the snug of your local in a roar, but, trust me, you're not Les Dawson.
- Brevity is not only the soul of wit, it's the secret of a good speech. Leave 'em wanting more. They want to get back to the drink and talking to their friends anyway.
- If the audience is there to listen, rather than enjoy itself, you're leaning against an open door. Just don't rush it; deliberately speak slowly, pause occasionally and drink plenty of fluids. No, not alcoholic! Oh, I don't know though, it depends on how it's going. . . .

And good luck – you're a brave little soldier.

Terry Wogan

Chapter 1 **Principles of communication**

Angela Hall and Peter McCrorie

Many readers of this book will have attended conferences and listened to doctors making presentations. Think about these presentations. Which ones were memorable and why?

Communication is, by definition, a two-way process – an interaction. Presentation tends to be one way only, so is there anything at all that we can take from research underlying communication and how people learn that is of any relevance to the topic of this book? Assuming that the intention of your presentation is to inform your audience, so that something is learned from you, what do we know in general about how people learn?

People learn best when [1]:

- They are motivated.
- They recognise their need to learn.
- The learning is relevant, in context and matches their needs.
- The aims of the learning are clear.
- They are actively involved.
- A variety of learning methods is used.
- It is enjoyable.

Presenting at meetings is not of course just about giving information ('I told them, therefore they know it') but about imparting it in such a way that people understand and take something away from it. Can we draw a parallel with the information-giving process between doctors and patients? There is in fact much evidence from research into medical communication showing that the following behaviours result in the effective transmission of information from doctor to patient [2]:

- Decide on the key information that the patient needs to understand.
- Signpost to the patient what you are going to discuss.
- Find out what the patient knows or understands already.

How to Present at Meetings, Third Edition. Edited by George M. Hall and Neville Robinson.
© 2012 George M. Hall and Neville Robinson. Published 2012 by John Wiley & Sons, Ltd.

- Make it manageable – divide it into chunks.
- Use clear, unambiguous language.
- Pace the information so that the patient does not feel overwhelmed.
- Check what the patient has understood.
- Invite questions.

Adopting these behaviours means that, as a doctor, you are doing your best to ensure that your patient both hears and understands what has been said.

What can we take from these two sets of principles that is directly relevant to giving presentations at meetings?

Preparation

Know your audience

Decide what it is about your topic that you want your audience to understand. The presenter is usually in the situation of knowing a lot more about the subject than many of the people in the audience. Find out about your audience. What is their level of knowledge likely to be? How many are likely to be there? The smaller the number, the greater the potential for interaction. Is the language in which you are giving your presentation your audience's first language? Regardless of first language, will your audience have a feel for the technical/medical/scientific terminology with which you are so familiar? Above all, avoid the temptation to try to impart more information than your audience can possibly assimilate. Message – keep it simple.

Don't let yourself get too anxious

Anxiety on the part of either the giver or receiver can act as a barrier to effective communication. Most experienced presenters will tell you that they are always anxious before starting their talk and this does not necessarily get better over time. It is normal and can be advantageous – a certain amount of adrenaline actually makes for a more exciting presentation. Lack of anxiety often results in the presentation appearing a bit flat. On the other hand, too much anxiety is a problem not only for the speaker but also for the audience. An audience can feel embarrassed and show more concern for the state of mind of the speaker than for what is being communicated. Sometimes deep-breathing exercises can help. Most people find that once they get started, anxiety drops to manageable levels. As with an examination, the worst time is just before you turn over the paper.

Rehearse your presentation

An important key to anxiety reduction is to know that you are properly prepared. Not only should you be sure about what you are going to say but how long it will take to say it. This means practising your presentation, preferably in front of colleagues whom you trust and who will give you constructive feedback. It is highly unprofessional to overrun and encroach on other speakers' time. A good chairperson will not permit this anyway, with the inevitable result that your talk will be incomplete or rushed at the end. Rehearsal is important.

Prepare prompt cards

What do you take in with you in the form of notes to your presentation? If all you do is read directly from a prepared script, there will be no effective communication with your audience. You might as well have distributed a photocopy of your talk and asked the audience to sit and read it.

Reading also removes any opportunity for eye contact, for judging how the presentation is being received, or for spontaneity. Have you ever laughed at a joke that has been read out to you? A far better solution is to use prompt cards. Prompt cards carry only the key points of your talk. They serve partly as an *aide memoire* and partly as a means of reducing the anxiety of drying up.

Check out the venue and equipment

Arrive at the venue early enough to check out the room size and layout, the location of light switches and the equipment you are intending to use. If you have opted for a PowerPoint presentation, check that the system is compatible with your computer/USB flash drive.

Always bring back-up overhead transparencies – just in case disaster strikes. Check that your slides/overheads are visible from the back of the hall. Be sure you know how to operate the equipment – computer, laser pointers, lectern layout, video recorders, etc. The audience will be irritated if you are apparently experimenting with your equipment at the start of your presentation.

Content

Say what you're going to say, say it and then say what you've said

All presentations should have a beginning, a middle and an end. First, you describe the purpose of the talk and the key areas you will be considering. Second, you deliver the main content of the talk. This should cover:

- Why the work was done.
- How it was done.
- What was found.
- What it means.

Finally, you should summarise what you have said in a clear and concise way. Don't worry about repeating yourself. Repetition aids understanding and learning.

Put your talk in context

It is often erroneously assumed that an audience understands the context of a presentation. An example will illustrate this. Try to memorise as many of the following statements as you can:

- A newspaper is better than a magazine.
- A seashore is a better place than the street.
- At first, it is better to run than to walk.
- You may have to try several times.
- It takes some skill but it's easy to learn.
- Even young children can enjoy it.
- Once successful, complications are minimal.
- Birds seldom get too close.
- Rain, however, soaks very fast.
- Too many people doing the same thing can also cause problems.
- One needs lots of room.
- If there are no complications, it can be very peaceful.
- A rock will serve as an anchor.
- If things break loose from it, however, you will not get a second chance.

It's hard, isn't it? Now reread the statements in the knowledge that the title (i.e. the context) of the exercise is 'making and flying a kite'. This time, you will find it easier to recall the statements. Although this example may seem a little unusual, there is much documented evidence in educational research showing that learners are often not able to relate new knowledge to whatever they already know about a certain subject. Having a context through which new information can be related to existing knowledge results in better memory recall [3]. It is also important to put your presentation into a more general context – how it relates to others speaking in the same session, the meeting or conference theme.

Delivery

Pretend you are on stage

Giving a talk is not unlike being on stage. First impressions matter, so do not shuffle, fidget, mumble or talk to the projector screen. You do not want the audience to be distracted from what you are saying by how you behave. Remember that your nonverbal communication is as important as the words that you use. Grab the attention of your audience right from the start; you can appeal to their curiosity, tell an anecdote, use a powerful and pertinent quote. Smile and look confident. Speak slowly and clearly and vary your tone of voice. Look around your audience as you talk. Catch their eyes and engage them by being enthusiastic, even passionate, about your subject.

Decide on your mode of delivery

The medium of presentation needs some careful thought. The obvious contenders are flipcharts, overheads, and PowerPoint presentations. Which is best for you? With which are you most comfortable? Which is the most impressive? Which best illustrates the material you wish to present? These are questions only you can answer. You must weigh up the pros and cons and make a decision.

Make your visual aids clear and simple

Just as doctors can reinforce the information they give to patients with written materials or simple diagrams or drawings, your visual aids should illuminate or illustrate your words. If you are showing a slide, for instance, it is enormously helpful to state what in general it is about as you show it. If your audience needs to read something on your slide or overhead, stay silent for a few seconds. You will be very familiar with your material but do not assume that your audience shares your understanding; for example, say what the 'x' and 'y' axes represent on a graph; explain the key to your histograms. We would probably all like a pound for every slide or overhead that we have been shown in a scientific presentation that is impossible to see or interpret, for which the presenter apologises to the audience. So why show it? Why not make a new slide that summarises the point that the original was attempting to make?

Consider varying the delivery mode

Attention span is limited, especially if your audience is sitting through a series of presentations. In a presentation lasting more than 15–20 minutes, it is worth thinking about switching modes of delivery – for instance, to use a video clip to illuminate a particular point that you wish to drive home. Think about the visual impact of being *shown* an operating technique, for instance, versus a verbal description of it, or a real patient describing a condition they suffer from, versus your description of what such a patient might say.

Don't go over the top

We have all been to presentations that were dazzling – dual projection, fancy animated PowerPoint slides, video clips, etc. However, have we remembered a thing about the content of these glitzy presentations? Probably not. What is crucial is not to allow the medium to overwhelm the message. It may seem an obvious point, but the greater the number of modes of delivery, the greater the risk of technical failure.

Don't be frightened of questions

What is unpredictable, and invokes much anxiety, is the prospect of being asked difficult or awkward questions at the end. This is dealt with in more detail in Chapter 10, but remember that there will always be questioners who are trying to score points, gain attention or display knowledge rather than genuinely trying to find out more about your work or ideas. The audience is usually aware of this and will be on your side. If you know that there are areas in your presentation that may confound or compromise some of the evidence that you are presenting, address these in the body of your talk to pre-empt obvious points of attack from questioners. Remember that good research provokes as many questions as it answers and occasionally a member of the audience will ask the question that you had not thought of that will trigger your next research proposal. Doctors should not pretend that they know the answer to a patient's question when they do not. Similarly, admit to your audience if you cannot answer one of its questions, agree to find out the answer and remember to follow it up. You can sometimes engage your audience more actively if you throw the question back.

Look out for nonverbal communication

How you check what the audience has understood from your talk is clearly difficult though not impossible. The questions that you are asked at the end of the talk may give you some insight into the level of comprehension. However, what does it mean if no questions are asked at all? What is conveyed to you nonverbally from the audience during your presentation may be just as revealing. Do people look interested or puzzled? How many have gone to sleep? How many are fidgeting or have actually left the room? If you spot any such behaviour, either bring your talk to a conclusion or do something to wake up the audience, such as asking a question or telling an amusing anecdote.

Conclusion

There is real satisfaction to be had from giving a presentation that is well thought out, properly rehearsed, and confidently and enthusiastically delivered. Indeed, anything less indicates lack of respect for your audience and will leave you feeling embarrassed and disinclined ever to repeat the experience. Abraham Lincoln said, memorably: 'If I had 6 hours to chop down a tree,

I should spend the first 4 hours sharpening the axe.' The message is clear. Your presentation will be great if your preparation has been thorough. Take heart from the experience of most presenters, which is that although they may feel very nervous beforehand, once started they actually enjoy the experience. There are few highs to be compared with knowing that your careful preparation paid off and you got it absolutely right.

Summary

- Presentation tends to be a one-way communication process.
- Prepare your presentation well by understanding your audience, rehearsing your presentation, preparing prompt cards, and checking the venue and equipment.
- Think of the content: describe the purpose of the talk, deliver the talk and summarise.
- The delivery of the presentation is important – think carefully about both verbal and nonverbal communication and visual aids.

References

1. Knowles M, 1990. *The Adult Learner, A Neglected Species.* Gulf Publishing Company, Houston.
2. Silverman J, Kurtz S, Draper J, 1998. *Skills for Communicating with Patients.* Radcliffe Medical Press, Oxford.
3. Schmidt H, 1993. Foundations of problem-based learning: some explanatory notes. *Medical Education,* **27**: 422–432.

Chapter 2 **Preparation of the talk**

Mal Morgan and George M. Hall

The medically qualified actor, Richard Leech, stated that lecturing is like acting, in that the object of both is to tell a tale to an audience, but that the former is more difficult because you have to write the script as well. Contrary to popular belief, good lecturers are not born with an innate talent to lecture, although some do have more confidence than others to speak in public; this is not synonymous with being able to deliver a good lecture. However, like everything else, it is a skill that can be learnt, just like inserting a central venous catheter. It requires practice, discipline and adherence to a reasonably strict set of guidelines.

The two basic tenets of a good lecture are meticulous preparation, which takes time, and rehearsal. How do you go about preparing a lecture?

The invitation

The first time you are invited to lecture will engender a number of emotions, pride, to why me?, to sheer terror. It is true to say that there are a minority of people who are quite unable to stand up and talk in front of an audience, and if you are one of these then say so immediately. The organisers of the meeting want and should get a prompt reply. Whether you accept will depend on: (a) the subject and whether it is in your area of expertise (if you are an obstetric anaesthetist, do not accept an invitation to talk on 'The History of Medieval Welsh Codpieces'); (b) whether you have sufficient time to prepare the talk (it always takes longer than you think). It is absolutely essential that you read the invitation carefully to establish the 'ground rules' before you accept. Always keep a copy of this letter.

If you have reason to believe that you are not the first choice for this lecture, then do not be put off. Here you have a real opportunity to shine and make

How to Present at Meetings, Third Edition. Edited by George M. Hall and Neville Robinson.
© 2012 George M. Hall and Neville Robinson. Published 2012 by John Wiley & Sons, Ltd.

a name for yourself. Lectures given under these circumstances can give your career a lot of impetus.

Having accepted, you must now establish from the organisers a number of facts.

Type of meeting

This should be obvious from the invitation, but it isn't always so. Is it a 'one off' guest lecture or is it part of a symposium? If the latter, ask for a copy of the programme so that you know who the other speakers are in your session. As the subjects are likely to be similar in your session, it is a good idea to contact the other speakers to find out what they are going to cover. Do not be put off if you are told, 'Oh, I haven't thought about it yet.' If it is a research meeting of a society, you are not usually invited, but rather told by someone that you are speaking. These societies usually have strict rules of presentation that must be observed.

Subject

If you are speaking at a symposium there is little leeway with regard to the subject, but if it is a guest lecture, then you can negotiate with the organiser. Establish whether they want a review of the topic, or some of your original research around which you can build up a story, or whether they just want a discussion on future developments. Very often they will leave the entire content to you and, on occasion, allow you to choose whatever subject you like. Under these circumstances you have no excuse whatsoever to deliver a poor lecture.

Timing

Again this should be obvious, but check, and also see if there will be time for questions. It is never acceptable to talk over your allotted time, but no one will ever complain if you finish a little early.

Abstract

Establish at this stage whether an abstract is required for the meeting and if so what is the deadline. As abstracts are often required several months in advance for major meetings, this usually precedes the start of preparation of your lecture and merely indicates that they are of little value. However, if you know an abstract is required, it should be delivered by the deadline (and might even persuade you to start on your talk much earlier); not to do so is unprofessional.

Audience

Basic to the preparation of any lecture is a knowledge of who the audience are likely to be. This gives you some idea of what 'level' to pitch the lecture; on the vast majority of occasions, of course, these are your peers and therefore there will be no problem. The great mistake is to misjudge your audience, which is not a fault confined to prime ministers. You will leave a very bad impression if you 'talk down' to an audience or, on the other hand, 'talk over their heads'. This is one of the most difficult aspects of lecturing and applies especially if there are lay people present. How to judge this will only come with experience, but a basic rule is not to try to impress the audience but rather to interest them. If you can do this, then they will be impressed, especially if you have been dealing with a difficult and complex topic.

It is also nice to know whether any eminent members of the profession and your speciality are going to be present, that is any 'heavies'. You should certainly not be put off by this, but in fact should feel proud that they have come to your talk. Contrary to popular belief, they are not there to shoot you down at the end of your talk; they have all been through what you have and the majority are extremely helpful and complimentary. If they think that you might have gone off the track somewhere, they will tell you politely and usually after question time to save embarrassing you. However, as you will certainly have prepared your talk properly, such a situation will not arise.

The number in the audience is irrelevant. You will do exactly the same amount of preparation and rehearsal for an audience of 10 or 1000.

Title

The only thing that an individual sees about a forthcoming lecture is the title, so some thought should be given to making it attractive. A teaching lecture requires a short, didactic title, while an eponymous lecture usually has an obscure title which attracts people out of curiosity if nothing else. Titles for guest lectures should be in plain English and simple. The philosophy of Richard Asher, one of the greatest medical writers, with regard to titles of papers applies just as well to a lecture. Which would attract the greatest audience 'A trial of 4,4-diethylhydroxybalderdashic acid in acute choryzal infections' or 'A new treatment for the common cold'?

Preparation

How often have you heard a conversation along the lines: 'I see you are lecturing at the Royal College on Friday' and the reply: 'Oh yes, I must get on and do something about that.' The latter person is lying. This is just to give a macho impression that this person can prepare a lecture in 3 or 4 days;

this is impossible, and in reality this person has been preparing it for months. Proper preparation is the basis of a good lecture and, just as a brilliant actor cannot compensate for a poor play, a skilled and experienced lecturer cannot compensate for a poorly prepared talk. It is obvious to the audience if the 'spade work' hasn't been done. Unfortunately, there is a tendency for lecturers to 'go off' as they get older and the reason for this is usually because they ignore the importance and time required for proper presentation. They have done it so often before that they think they can always do it with the minimum preparation.

A long-retired professor of surgery, and a superb lecturer, once said that in preparing a new lecture, it took 1 hour's preparation for 1 minute of lecture; he was not far wrong.

How long before the lecture should you start the preparation? In fact, you do so immediately you have accepted the invitation, however far in advance of the talk. Long before you put anything on paper, you start thinking about it and this is a vital part of the preparation. You think about the content during idle moments, on your way into work and on the way home. Something your colleagues say might trigger a thought process about your talk and you might get ideas while listening to a talk on a completely different subject, for example on a possible layout for the lecture. If you are wise you should jot these things down so that when you finally sit down to formally prepare the talk you will already have a small dossier on the subject. It is surprising how much useful information you already have towards your talk. Never be afraid to ask the advice of your colleagues on the content and layout of your proposed lecture. They will invariably give you useful and valuable advice.

So, how far in advance do you actually start preparation? The answer, as soon as possible, and would that we were all disciplined enough to do that. The aim should be to finish preparation at least 1 month before the date, including visual aids. It can then be filed away and looked at two or three times before the talk. There is still time to change things if necessary, although, if properly prepared, this will not be necessary.

The actual preparation of the lecture should follow a strict discipline. This is basically the same whether it is a 10-minute or a 50-minute talk.

Collection and selection of data

The first essential is to realise that you cannot cover everything that is known about the subject in one lecture and this particularly applies to the shorter presentations. You will already have given a lot of thought to this and the decision on what to select is entirely yours. You will base your selection on the duration of the talk, remembering that it is unprofessional to overrun your allotted time, and the audience. Even if there are 'heavies' in the audience, very few will know as much about the subject as you. Remember that your aim is to interest the audience. It is perfectly acceptable to explain at the beginning of longer talks that you are not going to talk about certain aspects of the subject.

Arrangement of data

You have been asked to talk because you are an expert in the field and therefore you have an immense amount of data on the subject. You have selected what you are going to say and you must now reveal this to the audience in a way that is easy to understand and assimilate.

Introduction

The length of the introduction will depend on the duration of the talk and the complexity of the subject. This can be the most difficult part of the talk and if you can introduce something controversial at this stage, so much the better. Do not be afraid to make the introduction simple, especially if there are lay people present; you do not want to lose the audience at this very early stage. Unless you are naturally amusing, it is wisest to avoid being funny. This applies especially to international meetings even if the same language is spoken in the respective countries.

Main message

The preparation of your talk will have largely taken place in the library, where you are surrounded by reference material, or in your office or at home. Your personal computer will have undoubtedly played a major part in your preparation, but you may not have journals on line. It is imperative that you read all the papers to which you refer and not just the summaries. When you have collated all your data, you should write the lecture (some will prefer a word processor) in the order in which you are going to give the talk. Always keep all the references that you have used.

When it comes to delivering the main message, then do so in a logical sequence, using plain English, and giving your supporting evidence. Take the trouble to explain your visual aids, which the audience are seeing for the first time.

Conclusions

At the end of your talk the audience will expect relevant conclusions and it is also sensible to make some suggestions as to where the future lies, if applicable. Remember that if your title asked a question, then the audience have a right to expect an answer.

When you have written the talk you should now make the appropriate visual aids, having already established with the organisers what equipment is available. The lecture and visual aids are then filed. Never throw them away; you never know if they will be useful again.

Rehearsal

This is absolutely mandatory. The rationale behind a rehearsal is:

- to time the lecture, especially the shorter ones;
- to assess the technique of delivery, where annoying mannerisms can be spotted and removed;
- to anticipate questions;
- to give confidence to the speaker.

For 10-minute talks to research societies, the rehearsal should be in front of your colleagues, which is never easy. This should be done a minimum of 2 weeks in advance so that there is still time to correct slides and iron out flaws in your delivery technique. For the longer talks you should sit with your manuscript and visual aids and go through the talk and slides and time how long it takes. You should do this several times before your talk and you should do it every time you are going to lecture, even if it is the same talk. When rehearsing in this way, always go through the slides as you would at the actual presentation.

Presentation

You are going to be nervous when you stand up in front of an audience to talk, particularly the first time. Although the more experienced lecturers may not give this impression, you can guarantee that there will be a degree of apprehension. Under no circumstances should you resort to pharmacological help to allay this apprehension. It might get less with time, but it will never entirely disappear.

Lectures should not be read. It gives the impression that you don't know your subject and also keeps your head down and encourages you to mumble. Your head must be up, talking to the back row and, in order to do this, you must know and have learned what to say. Use your visual aids as prompts. Turn to them to refresh yourself as to the next point, then turn back to talk to the audience. This means you must learn what you are going to say – actors do.

The only reason why people want to read the manuscript is because they are frightened they might forget to say something. This is totally irrelevant because nobody in the audience would know you were going to say it anyway. If you do suddenly remember that you were going to say something 5 minutes ago, ignore it; do not go back to it. This does not mean that you shouldn't have the full script available, and even refer to it very briefly from time to time, but the professional doesn't need one.

Visual aids

The most important thing to remember about visual aids is that they are aids. Very clever things can be done with them these days, but they must not be allowed to take over. Superb visual aids cannot compensate for poor content and delivery.

The vast majority of talks involve PowerPoint projection. Whatever you use, some basic points apply:

- Give the impression that you know your slides, so be confident and know what is coming next.
- Use all the information that is on the slide or it shouldn't be there.
- Disclose the information progressively.
- Never go back – rather use two slides.
- Do not use full sentences.
- Do not read everything that is on the slides.
- Never flash through slides.
- Do not leave slides up when you have finished talking about them; arrange your lecture so that this doesn't happen.
- Do not overcrowd slides; use more than one.
- Never borrow slides; always make your own.

Remember that lectures take time to prepare and if your preparation has been meticulous and you have rehearsed your talk with colleagues and sought their advice, the lecture really won't be a problem.

Summary

- The key to a good lecture is preparation and rehearsal.
- Check the content of the meeting at which you are going to talk, the subject and timing.
- Understand the audience in order to select the right level at which to pitch your presentation.
- Think carefully about the title and the content of your talk.
- Select and arrange information according to the audience and time given.
- Rehearsal is mandatory.

Chapter 3 **The three talks**

Mal Morgan and George M. Hall

Hospital medical practice would be regarded as strange by many people and particularly the treatment of emergency cases. The latter present many more problems than routine cases, yet they are largely cared for by the junior members of staff. The same applies to lecturing in the medical world. The shorter the talk, the harder it is to prepare and deliver. Yet the 5-minute talk is usually delegated to the most junior trainees, the 10–15-minute talk to specialist registrars, while the 45-minute lectures are the province of consultants.

There are no rules about lecturing, but a format has developed that has stood the test of time and it works. Talks of different lengths require slightly different techniques, but the general principles are the same.

General principles

- You are in a conservative profession so dress accordingly. A slipshod appearance equates to slipshod work in the minds of the audience.
- Never start a lecture with a slide. You are frightened because everyone is staring at you. Stare back, moving your head slightly from side to side. The audience have a right to see who is talking to them.
- After your introduction and the first slide comes up, the lights go down and should not come on again until you have finished. Conclude with the lights on.
- Speak to the audience, only turning to your slides to ensure that it is the correct one or to illustrate some point.
- Stand still when you are talking. Actors always like to deliver their lines while stationary.
- Talk at your normal rate. Radio newsreaders talk at about 120–133 words per minute. The rate of speaking of five subjects experienced in presenting

How to Present at Meetings, Third Edition. Edited by George M. Hall and Neville Robinson.
© 2012 George M. Hall and Neville Robinson. Published 2012 by John Wiley & Sons, Ltd.

papers and difficult material clearly varies from 106 to 158 words per minute. Never try to talk more quickly to get more information across.

- At international meetings it is a courtesy to talk more slowly. If there is simultaneous translation, provide a copy of exactly what you are going to say. As the spoken word is different from the written word, it will read terribly but translate perfectly.
- Do not try to be funny unless you are a natural, and smutty stories are strictly forbidden; you will always offend someone.
- When talking, punctuation is replaced by changes in the tone of voice, pauses and gestures. A monotonous voice with few pauses will guarantee that some members of the audience will go to sleep.
- Visual aids are an integral part of any good lecture and very few people have the gift of holding an audience's attention without them:
  Blackboard and chalk (whiteboard and pencil, etc.): This still has a place and can't be beaten when teaching small groups. The authors, however, have seen the late Professor Patrick Wall hold an audience of 400 enthralled using a blackboard. Flipcharts are dreadful.
  Overhead projector: Again, usually used as a teaching aid and has the advantage that the lecturer can face the audience at all times. The overheads require as much preparation and care as slides.
  PowerPoint: This has taken over from slides and, if used correctly, is extremely effective. However, computer-generated slides can and do go wrong. Your USB flash drive must be compatible with the hardware that is in use and you should have been told by the organisers what equipment they have. The biggest danger is that you are using the latest software, but the organisers are not. Great people (and the audience) have been embarrassed by having to wait 15 minutes or more before they have functioning visual aids. This problem can be avoided by sending the presentation to the organisers by e-mail several days before the meeting.
  Videos: These are only rarely needed to complement a lecture and, when indicated, can be a very worthwhile part of a PowerPoint presentation. However, they frequently go wrong. The video must be switched off immediately after your point has been made.
- Rehearse, rehearse, rehearse.

Day of the lecture

Despite your nerves, you must check a number of points when you arrive.

The chairman
Seek out the chairman and introduce yourself. You might know him/her, but he/she is unlikely to know you, especially when you are starting out in your

career. Chairmen get nervous too and want to know that their speakers are present.

The lectern

Look at this beforehand and familiarise yourself with the layout. Lecterns can vary considerably from being very simple to resembling a Boeing 747 cockpit. Ensure that you know how to call up your slides, especially the first one, and know how to go forwards and backwards and whether you, or the projectionist, controls the lights. A good chairman (see Chapter 12) will know what to do, but chairmen vary as well.

The microphone

The best are pinned to your clothing, which allows you some movement while talking without the sound level varying; fixed microphones have the disadvantage that you have to ensure that you are talking into it at roughly the same distance all the time, even when you turn to your slides. This is where PowerPoint projections have advantages. When you stand up on the podium, pin the microphone on yourself and do it quickly.

The pointer

This will either be something elongated (billiard cues are favourites) or, more often nowadays, a laser pointer (where the battery is usually on the verge of failing – check beforehand). Whatever the pointer, the technique of using it is the same. Always point to the aspect under discussion so that it is clear to the audience. Complicated illustrations can require a lot of 'pointing'. If you are worried about a tremor when using a laser pointer, then hold it in both hands while steadying yourself by leaning on the lectern. Remember to switch off the laser after making your point, as it is potentially dangerous to leave it on when you turn to face the audience as eyes can be damaged.

Once you are satisfied with all the above points, check them again.

The 5-minute talk

These are usually the province of the most junior members of the profession, who are told by their seniors that they are going to do it, and they have no say in the matter. Furthermore, the notice is usually short and you will be lucky if you have 2 weeks; 24 hours is not unusual.

Such talks usually involve case reports, or some aspect of an interesting case, with a mini review of the salient features. The fact that the time for preparation is short must not be used as an excuse for a slipshod presentation.

Presenting all the important features in 5 minutes is not easy and the use of visual aids will be limited:

- A PowerPoint presentation is unnecessary for this sort of talk.
- The overhead projector is useful for a 5-minute talk. Do not underestimate the value of overheads. They are used by the brilliant Professor Michael Sandel of Harvard whose superb lectures have been made into TV programmes. The overheads must be prepared in advance but do not overcrowd them. It is quite permissible to write them rather than get them typed. Make sure that they are in order and that they do not stick together. There must be a flat surface on which to place the overhead once it has been used and another on the other side of the projector for the ones you are going to use; do not confuse them. Practise with the overheads before your presentation so that delays are avoided. It is embarrassing to see people fumbling with their overheads during the talk. Some people like to reveal the points on the overheads one by one by covering them up with a piece of paper. This is not necessary and is often messy.
- If you are going to show radiographs make sure that you have them in your possession (there is a great tendency for them to go missing) and that you have a functioning viewing box.
- You might be presenting a patient; remember to explain everything to him/her. You must preserve their dignity at all times.
- Even though the notice might have been short, you should try to find time to rehearse; you can always find a colleague willing to spare a few minutes. Overrunning on such a short talk is indefensible.

The 15-minute talk

Such talks are usually the remit of more senior members of the trainee staff such as specialist registrars. You might be told you are doing this or be chosen by agreement.

Talks of this duration are usually a research presentation to a society and you will have been one of the workers involved in the project. This work might have been going on for a year or more. It would be unfair not to admit that these presentations cause more angst and stress than any other. Senior academic members of the profession will be present and you will be terrified that you might make a fool of yourself. However, remember that you have been working in the field for some time and you will know the subject intimately. There will be very few people present with such detailed knowledge. Conversely, of course, you are going to have to present your information in such a way that it is going to interest the vast majority of the audience, who will only have a passing acquaintance with the subject.

Putting facts that you know well to a general audience requires considerable skill.

There are a number of points to bear in mind when you have been chosen to give such a talk:

- A research society will probably have rules, for example nothing must be read. Know these rules.
- You have been chosen to present the results of research work that might have been going on for a year or more and involved several collaborators. You must not let them, or yourself, down, so preparation must be meticulous.
- You cannot get a year or more's research work into 15 minutes. Selection of data is therefore vital and you must decide with your co-workers what you want to get across; this will probably be only one major point. Do not try to give more information than anyone can assimilate in 15 minutes.
- The introduction must be brief and state why you did the work. Give enough information so that the audience knows how you did your measurements; things can be expanded during questions. In such a short talk you should use only your own original material and should not show slides of other people's work to illustrate a point.
- Do not be tempted to use too many slides. For a 10-minute talk, ten will be the maximum and six to eight are preferable.
- Speak at your normal rate. Do not be tempted to show an extra slide or two by talking more quickly. This never works.
- Rehearsal in front of colleagues is mandatory, including a final dress rehearsal. This is often stressful and you might feel foolish, but it must be done, and done in the way in which you are going to deliver your definitive talk. Rehearse as often as is necessary to get it perfect.

The 45-minute talk

These talks are usually given by the more senior members of the profession and are usually by invitation. The first time you are asked, the organisers might well be 'just trying you out'. A successful talk will usually mean that you get further invitations as word soon gets around; eventually you will become an established lecturer.

Once established, never lower your standards. Don't become blasé and think you can always deliver a good lecture. Preparation is everything and if you let this slip (usually because you are in a hurry), then a poor talk will result. Make sure that it is never you they are talking about when you hear 'he used to be a good lecturer'.

There are several types of 45-minute talks. For the teaching lecture, be enthusiastic and show the audience that you know the topic. Put yourself in the position of one of the audience and ask what you would want from a teaching lecture:

- The subject should be presented in a logical order, with clear headings and some discussion after each. Additional visual aids can be used to illustrate a point.
- Do not try to get too much in one lecture. If it is impossible to get over all the points, either decline the invitation or ask for two lectures.
- Deliver the lecture at such a speed that notes can be taken.
- Use clear visual aids.
- Keep the lecture up to date by reviewing it from time to time. You should not be giving the same talk in 10 years time – there will have been major changes.

At a symposium

You will have been invited to do this because you are well known in the field. Again, selection of data is critical and it is important to judge your audience correctly, which you should have done in advance. The subject of this type of lecture is usually chosen for you.

The guest lecture

Here the field is yours and you should establish from your host a rough idea of the subject matter. You have no excuse for not preparing a talk such as this properly, particularly if the subject is left entirely up to you.

The eponymous lecture

Usually given by the good and the great at the culmination of their career. These talks usually attract the most senior members of the speciality and frequently those from other disciplines; lay people often attend.

It is customary to say something about the person whose name is attached to the lecture, remembering that members of the family may be present. If possible try to say something that leads into the substance of your talk. These days, the latter does not have to relate to the interest of the person whose name you are honouring. Occasionally, eponymous lectures are given at the start of your career and this can certainly help your advancement 'up the ladder'.

Is it worth it?

This is a question often asked by those who have gone through the problems of preparing and delivering talks at important meetings. Some do not think it worthwhile and never present again. However, there is no doubt that the feelings engendered after you have delivered a well-received lecture are extremely pleasant and many revel in being the centre of attention in the immediate post-lecture period.

On the other hand, you might like to read the paper by Taggart and colleagues [1] before answering the question.

Summary

- Talks of different lengths require slightly different techniques but the general principles are the same.
- An overhead projector can be used for a 5-minute talk.
- For a 15-minute talk information must be brief and to the point. Eight to ten slides will suffice.
- There are several types of '45-minute' talks: the teaching lecture, at a symposium, the guest lecture and the eponymous lecture and you should prepare for each type accordingly.

Reference

1. Taggart P, Carruthers M, Somerville W, 1973. Electrocardiogram, plasma catecholamines and lipids, and their modification by oxprenolol when speaking before an audience. *Lancet*, **2**: 341–346.

Further reading

Whitwam J G. Spoken communication. *British Journal of Anaesthesia*, 1970; **42**: 768–778.

Chapter 4 **Visual aids**

George M. Hall

Visual aids are essential in medical presentations and much thought must be given to this part of the talk. Very few speakers can hold the attention of the audience for more than a few minutes without using slides. It is very difficult to convey information clearly without visual aids. An excellent lecture can be ruined by inappropriate and illegible slides, or technical problems when the local equipment refuses to project your version of PowerPoint. Good visual aids always enhance a presentation and their skilful use should be learnt at an early stage in a medical career. The basic aids are:

- board and coloured pens;
- flipchart;
- overhead projector and acetate sheets;
- video;
- slides.

The most commonly used visual aid is the slide projected from a PC. However, the other methods merit brief comments.

Board and coloured pens

The forerunner of this technique was the blackboard and coloured chalks. Unless you really wanted to be an artist or graphic designer and have the necessary talent, do not bother to consider this as a possible medium. I have seen brilliant displays with coloured pens by anatomists as they have slowly and patiently explained the development of an organ, but this is a dying art and far beyond mere mortals. Remember that most people cannot write on a board in a straight line.

How to Present at Meetings, Third Edition. Edited by George M. Hall and Neville Robinson.
© 2012 George M. Hall and Neville Robinson. Published 2012 by John Wiley & Sons, Ltd.

Flipcharts

These are best kept for those in medical management who wish to scribble two or three words on a large piece of paper before hurriedly covering it lest their illogical thinking is obvious to the audience. However, if you belong to the 'I love clinical governance' minority sect you may find a flipchart helpful in confusing the audience.

Overhead projector

The acetate sheets needed for this visual aid must be prepared just as rigorously as slides (see below). With the introduction of PowerPoint the overhead projector has become less popular but it is still useful for a brief, 5–10 minute, presentation.

Videos

Videos are occasionally valuable in demonstrating a new practical technique. It is essential to obtain expert help, often from the university or medical school audio-visual department, to ensure that the video is of high quality. Do not assume that, because you can film the family barbecue on a damp Sunday in Sidcup, you are a budding Scorsese. A good medical video needs to be made by a skilled professional.

Slides

The guidelines for the preparation of slides have been well known for many years and yet basic mistakes continue to be made. If you are a novice, seek help and advice from senior colleagues who are recognised for their presentational skills. In many medical schools the audio-visual department is very willing to give practical advice and even show examples of how not to do it. Remember that visual aids are used to add to the content of the talk and should not distract with garish colours, silly logos and sound effects suitable for children's television. The ready availability of computer software packages such as PowerPoint (Microsoft) means that it is easy to prepare clear slides. However, it is also possible to make a visual mess with this programme (see Chapter 6). Guidelines for slide preparation can be considered under the following headings:
• general format;
• text;
• figures;
• tables.

General format (see Box 4.1)

The key principle to remember is 'the fewer slides the better'. A problem with using programmes, such as PowerPoint, is that it is easy to present too many slides, so that the impression left with the audience may be literally that of a 'moving picture show' as slides flash by. The absolute maximum number of slides is one for each minute of the talk but a more sensible rate of projection is six slides per 10 minutes of talk.

A plain uncluttered appearance of the slide is necessary to emphasise the content. Avoid logos: most of the audience are not interested in where you work and know that they are attending the Third International Congress on Equine Euthanasia. Avoid frilly edges to the slide: the audience will think that you are a dress designer or worse, and avoid moving images, unless you want to ensure that the slide is not read.

The choice of colours is of great importance. It is traditional to use a light colour on a dark background, such as yellow or white on a blue background and many different shades of these colours are available. Although out of favour at present, a dark text on a light background works well. The original technique was to use black lettering on white (a positive slide) and this is useful in situations in which the light in the lecture room can only be partially dimmed. A more modern equivalent is to use black on a light grey background. Never use dark colours on a dark background – red on a dark blue background is a favourite combination and it is hopeless. Remember that the road signs in the UK are yellow on a dark green background or black on a white background because these combinations have been found to be the easiest to read. If you are unsure about the colours to use, let the Department of Transport be your guide.

If possible, try to keep all the slides in a horizontal orientation. Most slides are shown with the long axis horizontally and the short axis vertically (approximate proportions of 3:2). If you use slides with a vertical layout then you run the risk of losing the top or bottom of the slide as some lecture theatres cannot deal with this orientation. It is very irritating to see some of the slide projected on to the ceiling or floor.

Finally, use the same format for all the slides, that is the same colour combinations, typeface, layout, etc. If you want your presentation to be

---

Box 4.1 General format

The fewer slides the better
Plain uncluttered slides are easier to read
Choose colours carefully, avoid two dark colours
Keep to horizontal orientation
Use the same format for all slides – colour combinations, typeface and layout

---

Box 4.2 Text

Six lines preferable, never more than eight
Give key words on a single line
Select clear typeface
Avoid upper-case text (capital letters)
Align text from left, right margin is not justified

---

taken as a coherent talk then your slides must reflect this and be consistent. Do not insult the audience by presenting them with a jumble of slides, sometimes known as 'pick-and-mix' slides, which you have obviously used before for many different talks. Instead of listening to the content of the lecture, the audience will be wondering on whom you last inflicted that dreadful, rainbow-coloured, illegible slide.

Text (see Box 4.2)

The most common mistake is to try to present too much information on a single slide. Never use more than eight lines per slide and if at all possible stop at six lines. If necessary, divide the content between two slides rather than cram in extra lines. This is a fundamental rule of slide preparation and must never be broken.

Do not write in complete sentences, unless they are very short; just give the key words in a single line. It is always preferable to keep to a single line for each point that you are making: you lose impact by using two or, even worse, three lines. Select a clear uncluttered typeface that can be read easily and scan some of the newspapers to gain ideas about those typefaces that can be read best at a distance. Avoid upper-case text (capital letters) as this is more difficult to read quickly than lower-case text. If you wish to emphasise a point, underline the relevant word; a different typeface occasionally works but can distract from the rest of the slide. The text should be aligned from the left, with the right margin left unjustified.

The golden rule is to keep the slides simple and avoid detail. If you have to explain the layout of a slide to the audience then you have failed.

Figures (see Box 4.3)

There is considerable scope for making a mess when drawing figures for slides. The same general principles apply to figures as to the text: the colour combinations must be consistent throughout the presentation and it is essential to avoid overcrowding the figures. Because the editor of a journal insisted that you combine four small graphs into a single figure does not mean that you should inflict the same layout on the audience. The decision of the editor was

---

Box 4.3 Figures

One graph for each slide
Use different symbols for different lines and not different colours
Give indication of variability, if possible
Label axes horizontally
Avoid three-dimensional images

---

based on the need to save space in the journal; your objective is completely different – that of imparting information with clear, unambiguous slides, so the rule is one graph for one slide.

Complicated pie charts often look impressive in publications but are not suitable for slides because it is difficult for the audience to assimilate the information rapidly. It is preferable to use different symbols for different lines on a graph rather than different colours.

This avoids confusion where lines cross or disappear into overlapping mean values. Although it seems instinctive to consider different colours for different lines, this only works if the lines are well separated. If possible try to give an indication of the variability of the data, but look carefully to be certain that this does not make the slide messy and detract from the message. If necessary, you simply tell the audience that the data on the variability of the results are available and that they will have to trust your statistical analysis for the presentation. All labels should be written horizontally, abbreviated if necessary – unless you like inducing neck injuries in the audience – and should be self-explanatory. You undoubtedly remember whom groups 1–4 were, but most of the audience forgot 15 minutes ago, so label them appropriately – for example sober, mildly drunk, very drunk, and members of college council. Avoid whizzy three-dimensional options: in most instances they add nothing to the presentation and just tell the audience that you are an anorak who reads the software manual.

Tables (see Box 4.4)

Tables should only be used in slides if they are very simple, as it takes much longer to read a table than it does to 'read' the same information presented as a

---

Box 4.4 Tables

Tables must be very simple
Tables used for publication are usually not suitable for presentation
Alignment of columns is essential
Use explicit labels and give units of measurement

Table 4.1 24 hour means (SDs) for air pollutants ($\mu g/m^3$ except PM_{10} – ppb) and daily incidence of wheezy cases and controls

	Spring	Summer	Autumn	Winter	All seasons
Pollutant					
Ozone	46.3 (16.7)***	40.6 (13.3)***	22.0 (15.4)	22.3 (15.9)	32.7 (18.8)
SO_2	13.6 (11.5)***	14.7 (14.3)***	14.7 (13.4)	27.7 (24.3)	17.7 (17.5)
NO_2	41.7 (19.1)*	37.8 (14.4)***	46.0 (17.6)***	48.7 (17.4)	43.6 (17.6)
PM_{10}	23.5 (11.6)***	23.8 (10.8)***	19.7 (10.7)***	32.2 (20.1)	24.9 (14.6)
Benzene	2.54 (1.24)**	2.59 (1.33)	5.08 (4.22)	4.08 (2.56)	3.57 (2.83)
1,3-Butadiene	0.86 (0.55)**	1.02 (0.74)	1.82 (2.01)	1.33 (1.34)	1.26 (1.34)
cis-2-Butene	0.19 (0.09)	0.22 (0.10)	0.47 (0.46)**	0.31 (0.30)	0.30 (0.30)
n-Butane	6.12 (3.71)	6.39 (3.57)	13.00 (11.65)**	9.14 (7.53)	8.65 (7.85)
tr-2-Butene	0.40 (0.13)	0.43 (0.16)	0.77 (0.64)**	0.54 (0.42)	0.53 (0.42)
Ethene	5.27 (2.66)***	5.49 (2.82)***	11.68 (10.00)	10.80 (7.58)	8.29 (7.16)
Ethylbenzene	1.36 (0.67)*	1.44 (0.76)	3.18 (2.85)**	2.17 (1.63)	2.06 (1.89)
Ethyne	3.48 (1.92)**	3.18 (1.66)***	7.08 (6.24)	5.63 (2.68)	4.82 (3.94)
n-Heptane	0.30 (0.15)***	0.30 (0.15)***	0.63 (0.55)	0.52 (0.37)	0.44 (0.37)
n-Hexane	0.69 (0.47)**	0.76 (0.44)**	1.23 (1.04)	1.11 (0.85)	0.94 (0.77)

(Continued)

Table 4.1 (Continued)

	Spring	Summer	Autumn	Winter	All seasons
m-+p-Xylene	3.36 (1.74)*	3.62 (2.02)	8.07 (7.31)***	5.29 (4.22)	5.14 (4.86)
o-Xylene	1.38 (0.74)*	1.31 (0.64)*	3.20 (2.99)**	2.23 (1.71)	2.06 (1.95)
cis-2-Pentene	0.14 (0.07)	0.17 (0.99)	0.38 (0.20)***	0.22 (0.20)	0.22 (0.23)
iso-Pentane	6.59 (3.94)	7.67 (4.27)	11.93 (10.86)***	7.56 (7.30)	8.44 (7.41)
trans-2-Pentene	0.23 (0.13)	0.32 (0.19)	0.69 (0.66)***	0.40 (0.38)	0.41 (0.43)
me-Pentane	2.70 (1.47)*	2.93 (1.58)	5.47 (5.17)*	4.12 (3.56)	3.80 (3.48)
n-Pentane	1.32 (0.77)*	1.58 (0.91)	2.61 (2.19)**	1.79 (1.35)	1.82 (1.49)
Toluene	6.37 (3.27)*	6.92 (3.57)	14.00 (12.63)**	9.76 (7.99)	9.26 (8.39)
Ethane	5.15 (2.24)***	3.83 (1.76)***	6.69 (5.14)	7.88 (3.54)	5.88 (3.74)
Propane	2.36 (1.31)***	1.95 (0.99)***	4.02 (3.13)	4.58 (2.27)	3.22 (2.36)
Isoprene	0.26 (0.20)	0.60 (0.31)***	0.48 (0.41)**	0.30 (0.26)	0.41 (0.33)
Average HC	2.45 (1.19)*	2.40 (1.13)*	5.05 (4.25)*	3.75 (2.60)	3.47 (2.86)
Incidence					
All cases	3.2 (1.9)**	3.2 (2.8)**	5.1 (2.7)	4.5 (2.5)	4.0 (2.6)
Cases <2 years	2.0 (1.0)***	0.8 (1.1)***	2.3 (1.8)	2.0 (1.7)	1.6 (1.6)
Cases >2 years	2.1 (1.5)	2.3 (2.2)	2.8 (1.8)	2.5 (1.9)	2.4 (1.9)
All controls	63.5 (9.8)***	59.5 (10.1)	56.8 (9.9)	56.5 (9.2)	59.1 (10.1)

$p < 0.05$; ** $p < 0.01$; *** $p < 0.001$ v winter season.
SO_2: sulphur dioxide; NO_2: nitrogen dioxide; PM_{10}: small particulates with diameter <10 μm; Average HC: average of all 21 hydrocarbons.

Table 4.2 Estimated 8 hour TWA exposures* to MBT and its derivative by job and department title and by calendar period

| Department | Code | Jobs | | Applied to earlier periods | | | | |
			1955–60	1961–67	1968–77	1978–80	1981–81	1982–85
MBT solution	82936	Autoclave operator, dissolver bath operator, dayman	1.75	1.75	1.75	0.50	0.50	0.50
Bantex or Thiotax	99909	Centrifuge mill operator	4.25	4.25	4.25	1.75	1.75	1.75
"	"	Day bagging operator	4.25	4.25	4.25	4.25	0.88	0.88
"	"	Packing or flexible operator, precipitator operator	1.75	1.75	1.75	1.75	1.75	0.0
Pelleting	99905	Pellet operator	0.0	11.70	11.70	3.83	3.83	1.75
"	"	Day pack operator	0.0	11.70	11.70	2.33	2.33	1.75
Milling and blending	99980	Blending operator	1.95	1.95	1.95	0.64	3.24	3.24
Thiofide	82957	Senior operator, flexible operator	2.25	2.25	2.25	2.25	2.25	0.85
"	"	Bag flake operator, dayman	8.50	8.50	6.00	6.00	6.00	0.85
Thiurams	99970	Filtrate pellet operator	0.0	0.0	2.13	2.13	0.0	0.0
"	"	Dayman	0.0	0.0	6.50	6.50	0.0	0.0
All others	–	–	0.0	0.0	0.0	0.0	0.0	0.0

*The precision suggested by two places of decimals is spurious and should be ignored.

Table 4.3 Definitions

Knowledge	Specific information about a subject
Experience	Direct personal participation or observation
Competence	The condition of being capable, ability, the state of being legally competent or qualified

figure. Again the same basic principles apply: consistent colour combinations, a simple typeface and a clear layout. Alignment of the columns is essential in a table, otherwise the eye is drawn inevitably to the misalignment and obvious kinks. As for figures, use explicit labels and give units of measurement. It is almost always true to say that a table prepared for publication is totally unsuitable for presentation as a slide. For example, Tables 4.1 and 4.2 are taken from recent issues of the BMJ and must never be used as a slide. There is far too much information and most of it will be illegible when viewed from a distance. In marked contrast, tables suitable for slides are shown in Tables 4.3 and 4.4.

When all the slides have been prepared, go to a lecture theatre with a colleague and project them. Check very carefully for mistakes – they occur commonly and are more likely to be spotted by a colleague who has not seen the material before. Your colleague should sit in the back row of the lecture theatre to ensure that all the information can be seen easily. If it cannot, then you have to change the slide. It is sometimes hard to admit that your favourite slide is less than perfect, but it is important to find out well before the presentation. When all the slides are correct then you can start to go through the talk. As you rehearse check that the slides fulfil the basic functions list (see Chapter 2) to ensure that they develop a coherent story.

After that you are nearly ready for the presentation. There is still the small matter of rehearsal, rehearsal, and, when you think that the talk is polished, even more rehearsal.

Table 4.4 Distribution of responses by country

Country	Respondents (n)	Country	Respondents (n)
Austria	2	Latvia	1
Belgium	3	Lithuania	2
Bulgaria	2	Norway	4
Czech Republic	6	Portugal	4
Denmark	2	Russia	1

Summary

- Visual aids are essential when giving medical presentations.
- Only use board and coloured pens if you have the necessary talent; flipcharts are also not encouraged.
- Videos are occasionally valuable in demonstrating a new practical technique.
- Slides in PowerPoint are the most common form of visual aid used.
- Remember that the fewer slides used the better, keep them simple and make figures and tables easy to understand.

Chapter 5 **Poster displays**

Philip M. Sedgwick

What is a poster?

A poster is a visual and static display of your research project to potentially a large group of individuals at a conference or meeting. A poster is a combination of text and graphics. Posters allow personal interaction and discussion with, plus feedback from, 'interested' individuals. You may be required to stand by your poster at some point during the meeting in order to answer any questions that other participants may have. Recently, it has become popular for authors to provide a brief overview of their project via an oral presentation lasting two to three minutes. This will be done in front of your poster at a specified time in the conference, and may be followed by questions from interested readers. Posters have traditionally been used to communicate research. However, they have become a popular tool for presenting audit, plus a means of communicating research and experiences in disciplines including the social sciences and humanities.

There may be hundreds, or even thousands, of posters at a conference. Delegates may have been attracted to your poster by your abstract in the conference proceedings. However, you will also need to attract readers at the meeting. To do so, and then ensure that their interest is maintained, your poster must look interesting and be visually appealing.

The key to a successful poster is planning and development – a good poster is not constructed overnight. A poster will only provide a snapshot of your project – there simply is not enough room to present your work in the same amount of detail as in a journal article. You must choose what parts and key messages from your project you wish to communicate. Your poster must have a clear storyline; it should tell the reader what you did, why you did it, how you did it and the knowledge obtained. Make every effort to tell the reader why your project is important and why they should read your poster.

How to Present at Meetings, Third Edition. Edited by George M. Hall and Neville Robinson.
© 2012 George M. Hall and Neville Robinson. Published 2012 by John Wiley & Sons, Ltd.

Your poster must be understood with little, if any, difficulty. The poster must demonstrate clarity, succinctness, visual appeal but most of all it must be accessible. By keeping text to a minimum with a focus on the main points, it should be possible to read your poster in less than 10 minutes.

Constructing your poster

Identify your audience

Before you construct your poster, identify who your audience will be. Conferences are becoming increasingly multidisciplinary. Organisers therefore often request that posters are accessible not only to the specialist but also to the general professional audience.

Structure

Find out the allocated space for your poster. Size A0 (85 mm × 1189 mm) seems to be the most common format, either landscape or portrait. While this may seem to be a large amount of space, you must not cram it full of information. A poster only serves to provide a snapshot of your project.

It is essential that you structure your poster in a simple and logical way. The format of your poster may be dictated by conference organisers. A medical or scientific poster will typically have sections similar to a published journal article (see Figure 5.1), including title, aims, introduction, methods, results, discussion, conclusions, references and acknowledgments. It is suggested that you do not include an abstract, not least since space is limited, while the poster is a synopsis of your work anyway. However, a poster is not simply the sections of a journal article stuck on a large piece of paper. You cannot use the same detail as in a manuscript – posters have a different objective and you simply do not have the room. Note that the sections in Figure 5.1 are not necessarily the size they should appear on your poster - no doubt they will vary between posters.

By structuring your poster it will help you focus and synthesise your thoughts. Furthermore, and perhaps most importantly, it will help the reader easily establish exactly what you did. It really does not help if, for example, the aims are interwoven with your introduction or if the methods and results are combined.

Computer software

It has become popular to construct posters using computer software such as PowerPoint. You can then have your poster printed on the appropriate sized paper by a printing bureau. Alternatively, you could print your poster on

Figure 5.1 Suggested sections for a medical research poster. Your organisation may require you to adopt their corporate style, including the institution's logo. St George's University of London logo reproduced with permission.

numerous sheets of paper and attach to the posterboard on the day. However, this will not look professional and has limited visual appeal.

Poster orientation: portrait or landscape?

Portrait or landscape? Often it is your choice. If your poster is to be in landscape then it is recommended you have three columns, and two columns if in portrait. The sections should be read from top to bottom and then left to right. Numbering sections often helps the reader orientate themselves.

Title

The title should be succinct. If possible include the study design methodology used, such as double-blind controlled trial, questionnaire survey or qualitative study. Do not forget to include all of the authors and their affiliated institutions.

Main body of the text

- There is no way of estimating how much information you can include. It will, however, probably be less than you would like. A common pitfall is for authors to fill their poster with too much text with the result that it deters readers.

- The purpose of a poster is not to provide every single detail of your project. Establish the key take-home message(s) and present the necessary information to substantiate it.
- In the Introduction section give an overview of the most important literature.
- The Methods section provides insight to the process of how you conducted your project. Remember that readers will not have time to read a lot of technical detail – if they are interested then they can always ask you.
- The Results section should only contain the results from your project that corroborate your take-home message(s).
- Use the Discussion section to appraise the presented literature critically based on your results. Also outline the study limitations in this section.

Tables, diagrams, figures and graphics

Avoid excessive text in the Results section. Refer the reader to the bulk of your results presented either in tables or figures. Tables should not contain a lot of information. Remember you need only outline the key results or findings of your study. See Tables 4.1 and 4.2 for examples of the types of tables that are best avoided.

A figure such as a scatter plot can be useful to display complex information, for example the relationship between body mass index and blood pressure. Always remember to label your axes. Be careful of using figures excessively and/or unnecessarily. They may look appealing but might not add much information. For example, a pie chart can be useful to describe the distribution of ethnicity or biological sex. However, consider if the data could be more easily presented in the text or incorporated into a table, thereby taking up less valuable poster space.

Most posters will be read in less than 10 minutes. It is therefore essential that data presented in tables and figures is done clearly and effectively; otherwise the message will be misleading or confusing (references [1] and [2] give further guidance).

Diagrams are often a good way of communicating information. For example, a flowchart is useful for describing a clinical protocol. It is easier to describe physiological processes or anatomy using a diagram. Diagrams make your poster come alive.

Graphics or photographs are visually appealing. While they may not aid understanding or explain your results, they can serve to add aesthetic impact and make readers interested. Always acknowledge the source of graphics or photographs if you do not own the copyright. Ensure that any graphics or photographs are relevant, while not occupying too much space.

Always include a legend with your tables, diagrams and figures – legends should be concise while self-explanatory.

References

Between six and ten key references should suffice for a poster. Use Vancouver (i.e. number) rather than the Harvard (i.e. authors and date) style as Harvard can break the flow of reading.

If you have many references, the References section may occupy a lot of space. It would be acceptable to reduce font size (see below) for this section. Alternatively, you may consider excluding the title of the journal article and only provide the authors, journal, volume and page numbers. You might instead consider providing the Digital Object Identifier (DOI) for a journal article.

Font, font size and colour

- Use standard fonts, preferably Arial or Helvetica (sans serif).
- Make sure your poster can be read from a distance of one metre. The body of the text should be a minimum font size of 28 point, subheadings should be between 50 and 60 point, while the main title should be at least 80 point.
- Avoid typing in capital letters, underlining or shadowed text as they are difficult to read.
- Text is not easy to read if it is single spaced – use 1.5 or double spacing.
- Colours should be used to emphasise, differentiate and add interest. Use colours sparingly and with taste. Remember that your reader may be colour blind!
- Within each section, use black text on a white background within a black border. Set this against a pastel coloured background to make the poster easier to read and more appealing.
- Avoid using images for the background or textured backgrounds.

General advice

- There should be a storyline to your poster. Each section should be concise and self-contained, yet lead into the next section.
- Ensure your discussion and conclusions are based on your presented data, which in turn answer your original aims and ultimately reflect the title of your poster.
- Use straightforward language that facilitates understanding. Avoid complex jargon and excessive use of acronyms.

- Short sentences are the best. Long and complex sentences are difficult to understand and will only make readers abandon your poster.
- Consider using bullet points to simplify information, for example the aims of your project.
- Posters are primarily visual presentations so use strategies to attract readers. A poster should use tables, figures, graphs, pictures, etc., to tell the story of the study. Choose illustrations that are appropriate to the information you want to display.
- Balance the number of figures, graphics and tables against the amount of text.

Summary
- The poster provides a snapshot of your project.
- The key to a successful poster is planning and development.
- Choose your key take-home message and substantiate it.
- Your poster must have a storyline; tell the reader what you did, why you did it, how you did it and the knowledge obtained.
- It must be possible to read your poster in less than 10 minutes. Keep text to a minimum and focus on the main points.

Presenting your poster

You will need to interact and discuss your poster with interested individuals. Chapter 1, Principles of communication, Chapter 7, How to appear on stage, and Chapter 10, How to deal with questions, give valuable advice about presenting yourself and answering questions. You may even have to give a short oral presentation providing a brief overview of your project followed by questions. If so, it is recommended your presentation includes a summary of what you did, what you found and your key take-home message(s). Practise this short oral presentation in front of a mirror and time yourself – ensure that you look interested and that your presentation lasts between two and three minutes.

References

1. Altman D G, Bland J M, 1996. Presentation of numerical data. *British Medical Journal*, **312**: 572.
2. Freeman J, Walters S, Campbell M, 2008. *How to Display Data*. Wiley-Blackwell Publishing.

Chapter 6 **Data projection software: the hard facts**

William Harrop-Griffiths

Teaching tools have come and teaching tools have gone, but the temporal coincidence of the advent of both PowerPoint™ and the creation of the first company to produce data projectors in 1988 started a change in presentation techniques that will be with us forever. As chalk and blackboards, acetates and slides slipped quietly into the background, data projection and the software necessary to create the computer-generated slides used by the new generations of projectors came to the fore. After more than 20 years of experience with data projection, we should now be at a stage in which presenters are knowledgeable about how to get the best out of the presentation programs, the software is easy and intuitive to use, the connections between computer and projector are reliable, and the projectors themselves are not temperamental and never sit there stubbornly displaying a message that refuses to move from the flickering words: 'no input'. We are not yet at that stage, and I fear that it will be some years to come before we even approach that stage. There are still a multitude of mistakes to be made, problems to be encountered and frustrations to endure. This chapter hopes to steer you in the clear and quiet channel between the more obvious rocks that you can encounter on your journey towards presentation nirvana.

The basics

Hardware
You will need a computer, a data projector and the connections necessary to allow one to speak to the other. The vast majority of venues at which you will be asked to speak will provide you with a projector and a cable that ends in a standard, male, 15-hole VGA adaptor. This will almost certainly be connected to a computer that is a PC running a recent version of Microsoft™ PowerPoint™. The majority of presenters are happy to deliver up their USB

How to Present at Meetings, Third Edition. Edited by George M. Hall and Neville Robinson.
© 2012 George M. Hall and Neville Robinson. Published 2012 by John Wiley & Sons, Ltd.

flash drive containing their presentation to the organisers and then let them perform the transfer of the presentation file to the computer. However, a small but stubborn group of presenters insist on running the presentation off their own portable computer. If this is a PC, it is overwhelmingly likely to have its own, built-in female VGA adaptor that will mate happily with that on the end of the venue's projector's cable. If it is an Apple™ computer, it will not, and you will need to bring with you one of a bewildering variety of short connectors (sometimes incorrectly referred to as a 'dongle') that allow connection of the ports on the side of an Apple™ computer to a standard VGA cable. Every new Apple™ owner makes the mistake of forgetting to bring the short connector with them to the venue, but they tend to make this mistake only once.

Why would you want to bring your own computer with you to a venue when you could leave it safely at home and use the venue's facilities? There are several reasons. First and foremost, you can be absolutely certain that your presentation will run exactly the way you want it to when you have created it on your own computer and you have practised with that particular file on that particular computer. Although this is not of great significance if the presentation is relatively simple, it becomes more important if your presentation is complex, and includes sound, video and some of the cleverer, automated transitions between slides or graphic builds within slides. Another reason for using your own computer is that you can change your presentation even while waiting in the audience to be called up to the podium to give your talk, although I would not recommend this except in desperate circumstances. The main disadvantage of using your own computer is the transition period between you and the previous or subsequent speaker in which computers are nearly dropped, power leads are tied in knots, cables are disconnected and connected, microphones and laser pointers are exchanged, and the little clicky thing that allows you to bring the next slide up is lost. An experienced session chairman will draw the audience's attention away from the podium while you get your computer set up; the inexperienced chairman will allow the audience to focus on your difficulties and will cause a 30-second interregnum seem like a 10-minute hiatus.

Whether you use the venue's computer or your own, there is a *Griffiths's Golden Rule* that you should heed: get to the venue early and check that your presentation runs properly on the computer you are going to use; check every transition of the presentation and check that all the video and the sound files work properly. If you are using your own computer, insert the VGA cable into it and check that the computer talks to the projector properly. In the early days of data projection, you would often have to spend time adjusting the display settings in the computer to allow this liaison. Increasingly – but not always – computers self-adjust to data projection systems. However, occasionally, there is not a true meeting of electronic minds and you may need to make display adjustments or seek the advice of a nearby nerd or audiovisual technician. Having got the two electronic devices to talk to each other, disconnect and reconnect the VGA cable and see if it works a second time.

Griffiths's Golden Rule 1

Get to the venue early and check that your presentation file runs properly with the computer and projector you are going to use. Then check it again.

Software

PowerPoint™ is by far the most popular presentation software, and it has the great advantage of being genuinely ubiquitous, but it is not the only software available. Apple's Keynote™ is beloved by an increasing number of presenters because of its simplicity and versatile slide animations and transitions. Prezi™ (www.prezi.com) is a presentation concept that leaves behind the idea of slides, using one image as a form of memory map and causing the computer screen to seem to move around and zoom into and out of areas of the memory map. Whatever software you use, you should ensure that the computer that you are to use to run your presentation has the appropriate software to run it. This sounds a little obvious but many presenters have been caught out over the years. New versions of PowerPoint™ and Keynote™ are brought out by Microsoft™ and Apple™ on a regular basis for obvious commercial reasons. Although these new versions are always back-compatible, they are very often not forward-compatible. Let us take a theoretical presentation software package called Bulletlist. Bulletlist 2006 will almost certainly be able to play the previous versions of the software, Bulletlist 2002 and Bulletlist 2000, but if you have just bought the latest version (Bulletlist 2011) and take your presentation made with this software to a venue whose computer has only got Bulletlist 2006, it may not run. This brings us to Griffiths's Golden Rule 2.

Griffiths's Golden Rule 2

If you are not using your own computer for a presentation, take a version of your presentation file that is compatible with an older version of the presentation software than you have on your own computer – you cannot be sure that the venue will have the latest version.

If you obey Rule 2, you will take a file that runs with Bulletlist 2011 and one that runs with Bulletlist 2006. Most software packages have menu options that allow you to 'save as' or 'export' in previous software versions. In addition to this, Keynote™ allows you not only to save files compatible with previous software versions but also allows you to export Keynote files as PowerPoint™ files that can be run on Apple™ computers or PCs.

Getting the presentation file to the venue

In the early days of PowerPoint™, presentation files were small – often under 500 KB. With the advent of digital images and video clips, files have swollen rapidly, and a video-rich presentation file or set of files can easily exceed 100 MB. Gone are the days in which you could put two versions of your presentation on to a floppy disk and pop it in your pocket for the journey to the venue. With a capacity of only 1.4 MB, the floppy disk's days were numbered as a method of file transport. After a brief period in which CD-ROMs were the only way to carry large (up to 600 MB) files, the USB flash drive is now the popular porter of the presentation file. Often incorrectly called 'memory sticks' (this was a name used by Sony for a brand of non-USB flash memory cards), these portable, easily loseable and undoubtedly invaluable gizmos can now hold up to 256 GB of data – more than enough to carry a 90-minute feature film, let alone the presentation file to accompany a 45-minute lecture. However you plan to transfer your precious file to the venue, whether you attempt to email it in advance (often difficult now as even the more generous email providers limit the size of an attachment to 25 MB), carry it with you on a USB flash drive or on the hard drive of your portable computer, only the foolish would disobey Griffiths's Golden Rule 3: always carry a backup on a carefully virus-checked storage device.

> Griffiths's Golden Rule 3
>
> Always carry a backup of your presentation with you – and carry a backup of that backup too – and another one. You can't have too many backups.

The author's personal practice, borne of a longstanding obsessive–compulsive disorder and bitter personal experiences over two decades of looking daft in front of audiences because something has gone wrong with the technology, has led him to the following routine:

- Presentation created using the current version of Apple™ Keynote™.
- Copies made in previous versions of Keynote™ and as a PowerPoint™ file.

- Copies of each file kept on a portable computer and separately on a portable USB hard drive and USB flash disk.
- USB flash disk carried separately to computer and hard drive in case of theft.
- Copy of presentations stored on a cloud.

The use of the word 'cloud' may have confused some; let me explain. Cloud technology places a facility for data storage somewhere remote from your computer but linked to it via an Internet connection. You upload your files to the cloud and, when you want to use them, you can download them. Wherever you are, you can therefore access your files provided you can access the Internet. There are now hundreds of cloud providers, the most famous of which might be Google Documents™ and Apple's Mobile Me™. The beauty of this form of file security is that even if you, your computer, your hard drive and your flash disk all fall into a swimming pool on the way to the venue, thereby destroying all three versions of your files, you can still ask a friend at the venue to download a backup version of your file from your cloud. It is as near perfect security as you can get at the moment.

The clever bits

General advice

Presentation software packages can do some really clever things, and when you start using them, you will be tempted to explore some of the more complex technical crevices of the software. You will feel the need to use interesting and different fonts on complex backgrounds, animated transitions that involve rotating cubes or leaping flames, and slide builds in which words spin and cavort their way on to the slide accompanied by humorous sounds. My advice to you is to resist as best you can. Everyone who has wasted as many hours as I have creating complex presentations eventually comes round to the great truth encapsulated in both the 'KISS Principle' and Griffiths's Golden Rule 4: Keep It Simple, Stupid!

> Griffiths's Golden Rule 4
>
> Keep your presentations as simple as possible. Complexity only rarely enhances a presentation, and on-screen presentation software gymnastics are all too often more irritating than they are illuminative.

The following recommendations will keep you on the straight and narrow:
- Use a simple, clean font. Debate rages about whether serif fonts are easier to read when projected than sans-serif fonts. The author favours the sans-serif

Gills Sans	Keep it simple, stupid!
Helvetica	Keep it simple, stupid!
Arial	Keep it simple, stupid!
Times New Roman	Keep it simple, stupid!
Book Antiqua	Keep it simple, stupid!
Cambria	Keep it simple, stupid!
ITC Edwardian Script	*Keep it simple, stupid!*

Figure 6.1 Common fonts used in presentations.

fonts Gill Sans, Helvetica and Arial, in that order. If you like serif fonts, I would go for Times New Roman or Book Antiqua, although Cambria has a growing following. Avoid fonts such as ITC Edwardian at all costs (see Figure 6.1).

- Dark type on a light background projects well, as does light type on a dark background. Do not be tempted by coloured fonts and patterned backgrounds – their attraction fades very rapidly for the audience. Exercise caution in the use of reds and greens – there are more colour-blind people out there than you think.
- If you must use complex slide transitions to demonstrate the cleverness of both yourself and your chosen presentation package, then keep these to the minimum – one or two at the beginning or end of the talk.
- Only build slides (adding lines, bullet points or graphics to a slide) when you need to or if it makes things clearer for the audience. A 45-minute talk with every slide built bullet point by bullet point can get wearing.
- Graphic builds (where images or shapes are brought into the slide) can be very effective if used sparingly and with thought. Too many high-speed builds can become uncomfortably mesmeric.
- The best transition and the best build is called 'appear', in which the next slide of the next bullet point simply 'appears'. Seeing a word spiral down from the ether over two seconds is interesting once. Any more than this can evoke nausea.
- Slide builds accompanied by sounds are best avoided.
- Avoid 'busy slides', i.e. ones with too much content.
- Use a spell-checker – there is no excuse for 'typos'.

Images

The simultaneous development of both digital photography and the Internet has made countless millions of images available to the presenter. Images can be useful when explaining difficult concepts, and can add variety to your presentation. However, they can also be copyright protected, so you should exercise caution when using images and in particular when sharing copies of your presentation. If the image you have downloaded from the Internet has a watermark that indicates the owner of the image, this is a huge clue that you might perhaps be unwise to display it in public. High-quality images are very memory-hungry and the use of just a small number of these can swell your presentation file from manageably small to uncomfortably huge. Both PowerPoint™ and Keynote™ include ways of minimising the size of files by compressing images to a size that matches the resolution of the image to the capability of most data projectors.

Video and audio

Used wisely, both audio and video can greatly enhance presentations. Video of a sufficiently high quality to project well is very memory-hungry and can greatly add to the size of the presentation files. Video files used in Keynote™ are included in the presentation file. However, video files are not usually included in PowerPoint™ files. When creating the PowerPoint™ file, you effectively tell the presentation where in the computer the video file can be found. This simple fact has led to countless ruined presentations – either because the hapless presenters have forgotten to bring the video files with them on their USB flash drive or, even if they have, they have not been transferred on to the computer being used for the presentation or, even if they have, the presentation software cannot find them on the computer. Griffiths's Golden Rule 5 gives advice on how to avoid such disasters.

> Griffiths's Golden Rule 5
>
> When using audio or video files in PowerPoint™, keep the source files in the same folder as the PowerPoint™ file and put the whole folder on your media storage device, e.g. USB flash drive, when you go to the venue. Transfer the folder intact to the venue's computer and then obey Griffiths's Golden Rule 1.

Handouts and copies of presentations

Both PowerPoint™ and Keynote™ allow the printing of handouts, these most commonly being copies of the slides with or without space for members of the audience to make notes, with the presenter being able to decide how many slides should be printed on each side of paper. Another way of providing members of the audience with copies of your presentation, and one that avoids using paper and ink, is to make the whole presentation available either to the organisers of the meeting, who in turn can disseminate the presentation to audience members, or to individuals who request a copy. Small presentation files can be emailed, but if the file is large a version can be uploaded to a publicly accessible part of a cloud storage system. If you are reluctant to give people open access to the whole of your presentation file, you can export the presentation as a movie, which makes it hard (although not impossible) to copy sections or, if you have a working knowledge and full copy of Adobe Acrobat, as a Portable Document File (pdf), which cannot be copied, pasted or printed.

More advanced stuff

Presentation packages and modern computers allow the projection of one image on to the screen for the audience and another on to the small 'slave screen' or portable computer screen that the presenter can see – this is often called the 'presenter view'. It can show you a timer to allow you to pace your talk accurately, the next slide so that you know what is coming up and your personal notes (Figure 6.2). The use of this depends upon the computer being able to support 'dual displays'. The vast majority of recently manufactured computers can do this but difficulties can still be encountered, so make sure that the correct displays are projected for the audience and you (see Griffiths's Golden Rule 1).

There are few things more irritating than the speaker who mistimes his presentation and ends up skipping through slides to make up time. Experience

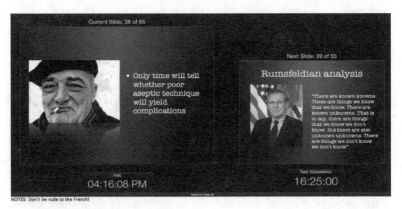

Figure 6.2 Presenter view (from Apple™ Keynote™ 2009).

Regional anaesthesia

- Rapid onset
- Prolonged duration
- 100% success rate
- Safe
- Fun

Figure 6.3 Action button (bottom right) allowing hyperlink to other slides in Microsoft™ PowerPoint™ 2008 for Mac.

and practice allow you to avoid this error, but sometimes the speakers before you in a session overrun horribly and you find yourself with much less time than you thought for your presentation. There is a way to make your talk flexible in terms of the number of slides that you show. You can insert visible or invisible hyperlink buttons (in PowerPoint™: Action Buttons) on slides that will link directly to other slides, thereby shortening the presentation without having to go through the slides one by one. A slight move of the mouse on the podium, a discreet click of the left button and you can bypass slides without any member of the audience being any wiser. Hyperlinks like this can also be used in interactive presentations to give audience members the choice of which of a list of topics you will cover next (Figure 6.3).

Closing comments

Computer-generated slide shows can enhance good presentations but they cannot make a bad speaker into a good one; good presentations are given by the speakers themselves, not by the computer and the data projector. Producing good PowerPoint™ or Keynote™ presentations takes time, experience and care. Simplicity is the watchword unless you are very experienced, very confident and very brave. When I look back on the presentations that I have really enjoyed, I remember the speaker and not the slides. Computer software is an adjunct to a quality presentation, not a substitute for it. Having said all this, there is a lot of fun to be had with presentation packages and their wise use can help even good speakers put over important points to the audience in a better and more comprehensible way.

Chapter 7 **How to appear on stage**

Alan Maryon-Davis

So you have worked hard on your presentation. You've honed it down to the key points. You've sorted out a few jokes. You've got great graphics. And you've timed it to a tee. In short, you've done about as much with it as you can, and as talks go, it's not at all bad.

But what about you yourself? How will you come across? Many a potentially excellent talk has been scuppered by inept presenting. We've all had to endure speakers who can't be heard, or who look all wrong, or who display some thoroughly irritating mannerism that completely distracts from what they're trying to get across.

How can you avoid such pitfalls? Better still, how can you appear confident and impressive on stage? Perhaps more realistically, how can you at least make sure that you don't get in the way of your own presentation?

Here are a few basic tips – most of which I have to confess I learnt the hard way – to help you avoid the likeliest own-goals.

Get there early

The first piece of advice is: make sure you arrive in plenty of time. We've all seen the consequences of turning up at the last minute. The chairperson looks anxiously at the clock, wondering whether to bring the coffee break forward. Suddenly there's a kerfuffle at the back of the hall as the speaker bursts in, rushes on to the stage, scrabbles around trying to load their talk on to the laptop and generally disrupts the entire proceedings.

You can avoid all that by getting there early. There are several advantages:

- It gives you time to load up your presentation before the meeting starts or during the break.
- It gives you an opportunity to pick up the 'feel' of the meeting and any issues that may have a bearing on your talk.

How to Present at Meetings, Third Edition. Edited by George M. Hall and Neville Robinson.
© 2012 George M. Hall and Neville Robinson. Published 2012 by John Wiley & Sons, Ltd.

- It allows you time to familiarise yourself with the stage set-up, podium, panel table, microphones and projection gear.
- It focuses your mind on the task ahead.
- It helps to calm your nerves and those of the organisers.

Sounds OK?

Grappling with an unfamiliar sound system is a classic elephant trap for hapless speakers. The usual disasters are failing to switch on the microphone, failing to make sure that it's pointing in the right direction, constantly clunking the lead or speaking so closely that you sound like a Dalek with laryngitis in a thunderstorm.

Spend a few minutes before your session starts to do a sound check – and if necessary make a few adjustments. If you're using a microphone on a stand – either a floor-stand, table-stand or fixed to the podium – adjust it so that it's pointing at your mouth, but is positioned slightly to one side of the direct line of fire of your breath as you speak. This is to avoid 'popping' – those periodic explosions accompanying every 'P' that punctuates a presentation. The microphone should be about 6 inches (15 cm) from your mouth and on the side nearer the screen, because if you happen to turn your head away from it, to look at the screen for example, your voice may disappear. To check the set-up, say a few words. Instead of the time-worn 'testing, one, two, three, testing', I would recommend 'Peter Piper picked a peck of pickled pepper' to sort out the pops from the snaps and crackles.

The lapel microphone may be a marvel of miniaturisation, but it can cause tons of trouble. First, there's the agony of where to clip it – a particular challenge for presenters without lapels. Women often find themselves in this awkward situation – and occasionally have to resort to holding the thing in position. With a radio microphone, the box of works can provide an even more difficult problem. If you have no pocket handy, you should be able to rest it on the podium. However, if there is no podium, or if you're standing at the overhead projector, you could find yourself with both hands full. Then there is the pitfall of failing to disconnect yourself at the end of your talk. This can either result in half your apparel being yanked away as you attempt to leave the podium or, with a radio mike, the much more disastrous consequence of inadvertently leaving the thing switched on and accidentally telling the world what you really thought of the questions you'd just been asked.

Looking good

Half the battle with successful presenting is to look good. By that I don't mean you have to don your best Armani – I mean looking self-assured and confident, knowing how to stand and move and generally having poise and style. If you appear to be comfortably in command of the situation it will help people focus more on what you have to say rather than the struggle you're having saying it.

As far as dress is concerned, this clearly depends on the type of meeting. What would be appropriate for a small informal lunchtime session for GPs might not be at all right for an international conference. My advice is to try to strike a balance between what you perceive is expected by the organisers and what you feel comfortable in. If there is a golden rule, I would say it's not to wear anything that either distracts or detracts from the message or impression you want to put across. So, fight temptation and leave that favourite ultra-loud tie or those knock-'em-dead sparklers firmly at home.

Standing and moving

It was once rather unfairly observed of the accident-prone US ex-President Gerald Ford that he couldn't walk down stairs and chew gum at the same time. Certainly many speakers do develop acute dystaxia when they get up on stage and have to cope with talking, following their notes, changing slides and pointing at things on the screen, all more-or-less simultaneously.

Good preparation and rehearsal can prevent most difficulties in this respect. I've already mentioned being familiar with the set-up, so that you know exactly which buttons to press. It also pays to have your notes (if you have any) clearly page-numbered, with bold headings, so that you can quickly navigate your way through them and instantly find your place again when you look up at your audience. They should also have clear prompts to cue each slide. If your talk is on PowerPoint or similar presentation software, you can include notes in the printout.

As soon as you hear yourself being introduced, go straight into presenter mode and walk confidently up those steps, smiling at the chairperson who hopefully has said a few nice things about you. When you reach your position, place your notes, check the microphone, smile at the audience and launch forth.

If you're using PowerPoint, the chances are you'll be speaking from the podium. Most speakers find the podium quite a comfort. Not only does it conveniently hold your notes, but it also gives you something to lean on in a casual, relaxed fashion, emanating calm professionalism. It's also a shield that you can literally and metaphorically hide behind, so that you don't feel so exposed.

However, others regard the podium as a millstone, encumbering their performance. They much prefer the freedom to move about, made possible either by a hand-held or radio microphone or a very loud voice. This provides a great opportunity to be more expressive, engaging and even dramatic. Be careful, however, not to overdo it. Too much strutting and fretting can distract from what you're trying to communicate.

Further points to watch when presenting with PowerPoint slides:

- Use the laptop screen as your prompt rather than the projection screen. That way you'll be facing the audience rather than the screen and it will be easier for you to maintain your eye contact. It's usually safe to assume that whatever's on the laptop will also be on the big screen.
- With an infrared pointer, use it sparingly – too much waving about is irritating. Also, avoid pointing at the audience – health and safety. If there's no infrared pointer to hand, you can use the arrow and touchpad, although it doesn't show up very well from the back of the hall.

How to speak

The key points are:

- Be audible. If you can't be heard, your words are wasted.
- Be intelligible. If your words can't be understood, the audience is wasted.
- Be engaging. If you don't hold the audience's attention, your slot in the programme is wasted.

Therefore, don't mumble. Don't speak in a monotone. Keep your chin up and project your voice to the back of the room.

Preferably use brief notes or your slides as a prompt rather than reading word-for-word from a full text. Leave plenty of pauses, especially after making a key point. It gives the audience a chance to take things in properly and you a chance to catch your breath.

Sound and look enthusiastic, or at least interested in your own talk. Nothing turns off an audience more swiftly than a speaker who emanates utter boredom and would clearly rather be somewhere else. If you don't look as though you believe in what you're saying, nobody else will.

On the other hand, don't swing too far in the other direction. Stressing every other word can be very wearing, a sing-song inflection can be thoroughly irritating and an overindulgence in arm-waving an exercise in distraction. So, plenty of enthusiasm, commitment, passion even – but not at the cost of losing the message.

Eye contact

It is important to get the eye contact right from the outset – it makes a big difference to how well you engage your audience. Here are a few tips:

- Don't just talk to your notes or the screen.
- Don't stare at the floor, ceiling, clock or out of the window.

- Don't just address the front row or two. The rest of the audience will feel excluded.
- Don't fix your gaze too much on someone who seems to be paying attention. You may lose the only friend you have.
- Do engage with all parts of the auditorium – middle, front, back, left and right – so that you draw the whole audience into your circle of confidence.

And finally . . . a word about coping with nerves

You may have done all the right things – carefully prepared your talk, rehearsed a few times in front of your colleagues, arrived at the venue early, checked all the systems – and still find that you're a bag of nerves as you wait to be called up on stage. What can you do to restore inner calm?

I wish I knew. I still have this problem to some extent after many years of appearing on stage, not only as an invited speaker but also as a founder member of the humorous singing group Instant Sunshine. Of course, there are all those tips about relaxation – deep breathing, imagining waves lapping on the shore, alternately tensing and relaxing your muscles, reciting a silent mantra. However, you're probably as unconvinced about all that as I am.

My advice is to just do it. Throw yourself into it. Ride the tiger. Harness the adrenaline to give your talk that vital bit of edge. The chances are you won't be looking anything like as nervous as you feel. Notwithstanding what I've just said, there is light at the end of the tunnel. It actually does get easier with practice.

Summary

- Make sure you arrive in plenty of time.
- If you can, pre-load your presentation and do a sound check.
- When speaking, be audible, intelligible and engaging.
- Maintain eye contact with the audience.
- Look and sound confident and relaxed – even if you aren't.

Chapter 8 **How to sell a message**

Martin Godfrey

Having a message and then selling it are central to the process of getting your point across – surely the main aim of any presentation. This chapter will help you to identify your messages, create them succinctly and get them across effectively.

Unfortunately the word 'message', used in the context of a meeting, doesn't usually do much for the average medic. It conjures up a variety of unappealing mental pictures, ranging from the archetypal Armani-suited marketing man spinning a story for some corporate seminar to the American evangelist proselytising to a football stadium of believers. Surely medics don't have messages; they have ideas or facts or data or something much less commercial.

However, I can reassure you: messages are OK. Messages are what you need to communicate effectively. In fact, no successful speaker or factual writer has ever gone very far without consciously or unconsciously being very good at creating messages and selling them. All the best politicians, journalists, business leaders, professors, dictators, etc., sell messages as a central part of what they know they have to do.

So let's start with the message. Before you do anything else in preparing for your presentation you must be clear about your messages. Use them to create a skeleton on which the rest can hang.

What is a message? A message is a simple statement of the main thing or things you want to say. It is, in effect, a succinct summary of the point you are making.

At their best, messages become virtual slogans: 'Vote Conservative' or 'Boris Johnson for Mayor'. They can be longer and do not necessarily have to appear as such in your presentation – they are merely what you would want to be left with if the whole thing was distilled down to a complete minimum. So a message might be: 'The Conservative party stands for law and order' or 'Boris Johnson will not nationalise the Underground'. Try not to overcomplicate.

How to Present at Meetings, Third Edition. Edited by George M. Hall and Neville Robinson.
© 2012 George M. Hall and Neville Robinson. Published 2012 by John Wiley & Sons, Ltd.

Journalists are trained to try to put their main messages into the 'intro-duction' – the first paragraph – of their news article. Since they have to make sense grammatically, these introductions tend to be a little longer than the raw message. However, the process of arriving at the gist of what they want to say can be used by anyone trying to cut through large amounts of verbiage to reach the key point underneath.

One useful tip to do this is to imagine you are walking down the street and you see your mother just getting on to a bus. You have something important to tell her, but the bus is moving off and thus you have only seconds to summarise what you want to say as you run breathlessly behind her. It's that sound-bite, that 'in a nutshell sentence', that will give you your main message should you be uncertain of its real nature.

How many messages? As a general rule, it is best not to have too many messages in a presentation. People can easily get lost if you are trying to say too much. The old adage 'keep it simple, stupid' is a good one to remember.

Therefore, have one or, at the most, two or three key messages – never more. If you feel you need to use more, you will probably find that many of the others are merely subsidiary to those initial key messages and can be developed as supporting points. If you still have more, then make two presentations.

Now you have your key messages, how are you going to sell them? First, you have to really understand your audience. Put yourself in their shoes and ask yourself the following questions as if you were being presented to by yourself:

- How will your ideas help me?
- What are the facts and where are the snags?
- Do I agree or disagree?
- What are my needs?

One of the great insights about effective presenting is that if you are really going to sell to your audience they must connect with the benefits of what you are selling. You must understand their individual needs and tailor your message-sell accordingly. For example, if you are selling a Porsche you should understand that the needs of most of those buying it will revolve around getting from London to Manchester as fast and with as much excitement as possible. They are not that interested in whether the car has side impact safety features or a 3-year warranty. Your message is that the Porsche you are selling is the fastest and most exciting car on the road. Selling it as the safest car on the road might equally be true, but it isn't what they want to hear – it's not what they need. Understand your audience's needs and address them directly.

Let's go back to the Conservatives. You are selling the message that the Conservative party is the party of law and order and you are presenting to a group of policemen. What they need is to have a party that will support them in doing their job. What they want is more policemen, better pay and a judiciary that has the power to convict.

What if the audience is made up entirely of medical students? They might simply want more policemen on the beat, more neighbourhood watch schemes and similar things. You can just imagine how difficult it might be to sell such a message to a group of students. They are suspicious, and law and order is not necessarily something that medical school students really think should be increased. They will more than likely be suspicious and only vaguely in touch with their own needs in this area. That's where the next trick to effective message-selling comes in. Don't sell *features*, sell *benefits*.

More policemen is a feature; fewer manpower shortages and thus less stress is the benefit to the policeman or woman. More beat policemen is a feature; more manpower to prevent burglaries around the halls of residence is a benefit. A 4-litre engine is a feature; 0–60 mph in 3.5 seconds is a benefit.

In other words, people buy solutions not things or services. A man who goes into a DIY store looking for a 1.5-cm diameter drill bit may not know it, but in reality what he is buying is a 1.5-cm hole. Thus, we have clear, simple messages, an understanding of the audience's needs and a desire to sell benefits, not features. How do you put all that together into a winning presentation?

No two presentations are the same, but there are some basics that you should attempt to ensure are covered:

- Introduce the presentation – highlight your key message(s) and ensure your audience is left with a clear idea of how you are going to address the topic. A map of your presentation is very useful here. Return to it frequently so your audience doesn't lose its way and get bored.
- Follow a presentation process. The classic method is first to analyse where you are, discuss where you want to be, outline the options and then deliver your chosen solution.
- Don't have too much verbiage on the slides. Your slides are effectively just wallpaper allowing you to highlight certain key points. Never have more than three words per bullet point and try to include lots of pictures.
- Make sure the benefits you are highlighting are clearly shown.
- Always summarise (in fact it is a good idea to summarise regularly through-out the presentation) and ensure your key messages are all in there.
- Ask your audience directly if they got the message. If you discover they haven't understood, let alone bought, the message then at least you have one last chance to get things right.

Lastly, a few words on presentation style. A great presentation can be lost if the presenter is not interacting with the audience, while a poor presentation can become a great one with an engaged audience.

Actors are often taught that to really interact with an audience they need to demonstrate a level of emotion and animation. To help analyse this emotional element, a ladder of seven emotional presentation styles was developed by a French actor in the 1960s:

- Level one: *Total exhaustion.*
- Level two: *The Californian.* Very relaxed, very friendly, but to the point. This style puts your audience at their ease and allows you to appear confident and unthreatening.
- Level three: *The stage manager.* This alludes to the neutral figures in black outfits who walk briskly on to the stage, move a piece of furniture then walk off again. They show neutral emotion. This is the state in which most people present and not surprisingly they do not succeed in connecting with their audience. Typically the presenter speaks in a monotone with an unemotional voice with few movements of any kind.
- Level four: *The director.* Animated, direct and sure-footed. Probably the ideal presentation style. The presenter feels as if he or she is in command of the room, looking at each member of the audience as he/she makes a point and only moving eye contact once the point has been made.
- Level five: *There may be a bomb in the room.* Very high energy, but usually too much for a normal presentation.
- Level six: *We found the bomb.* High, negative energy levels.
- Level seven: *The nervous breakdown.*

Always try to be in either the Californian or the director mode – years of practice has shown that these styles work. Don't forget to be positive and interested, ensuring that there is plenty of inflection in your voice. When you get to your key messages, try pausing to heighten the level of interest; emphasise them and, if necessary, repeat them to ensure you get the point across. Also remember to really feel interested in what you are saying. This may sound fundamental, but it is amazing how dislocated many of us become when we are having to present. If you aren't showing interest, it's certain none of your audience will be!

In summary, then, successfully selling messages in a presentation involves the development of a very few simple messages: understanding the audience's needs, selling benefits, not features, and ensuring (through practice) the correct projection of emotion and interest.

Summary

- Be clear about what your messages are and try to keep them simple.
- Only have two or three key messages in your presentation.

- Ensure that the audience understands the benefits of the messages.
- Maintain the right projection of emotion and interest.

Further reading

Fisher R, Ury W, Patton B. *Getting to Yes.* Century Business Books, London, 1991.
Kelcher M. *Better Communication Skills for Work.* BBC Books, London, 1992.
Senge P M. *The Fifth Discipline: The Art and Practice of the Learning Organisation.* Century Business Books, London, 1990.

Chapter 9 **How to present a talk**

Charlotte Green

For a lecture to be successful it is essential to engage the interest of your audience. The aim is to catch their attention, share your enthusiasm for the subject with them and, ideally, enlighten and entertain them.

This may be an apocryphal story, but I have heard tell of a lecture given at Oxford some years ago in a cramped and overcrowded room. Some people had to sit or even lie on the floor. The day was hot and the lecturer uninspiring; one student fell asleep and began to snore. The lecture was so stultifyingly boring that he continued to snore, uninterrupted, until everybody had filed out. Obviously, a less than memorable talk!

In order to interact with your audience and elicit a favourable response from them it's helpful to smile, look friendly and make eye contact. The latter should be fleeting and random; don't become fixated on the first friendly, responsive face you see, tempting as this may be if you are feeling nervous. It begins to look slightly peculiar if you return again and again to the same person and they may well start to feel distinctly uncomfortable. Equally, don't get downhearted if you appear to be getting very little response from your audience; it could just be the way their faces naturally settle when they're concentrating! When I take part in The News Quiz, which is a lighthearted and satirical look at the week's news on Radio 4, I've learned to adopt an attitude of what I call 'creative indifference'. Inevitably, my eye will fall on someone in the audience who steadfastly refuses to laugh and persists in looking grumpy and disgruntled. The best way to deal with this is to mentally shrug the shoulders and move on, concentrating on where the biggest laughs are coming from.

How to Present at Meetings, Third Edition. Edited by George M. Hall and Neville Robinson.
© 2012 George M. Hall and Neville Robinson. Published 2012 by John Wiley & Sons, Ltd.

Style of language

The late Bernard Levin used to write articles for *The Times*, comprising just one sentence. It was logical in its construction, embellished with umpteen dependent clauses and baroque phrases, but extremely difficult to follow, particularly if read out loud. At the other extreme, I have heard of someone who, facing a challenge to explain a statement in words of one syllable, did just that. The resulting paragraph was quite clear but very limited in its vocabulary and range of argument.

Aim for brevity, clarity and succinctness. It's always best to avoid long-windedness or 'gas-bag' English, such as 'alternative dentition' for false teeth or 'at this moment in time' for now. Simple yet vivid words will convey your meaning perfectly well. Avoid made up words that are a conflation of two existing words – it's amazing how many people say 'irregardless' when they mean regardless or irrespective. My favourite comes from President Bush, who was asked to describe the situation in Baghdad. He seemed to be momentarily stumped but eventually came up with the immortal line 'conditions there are horrocious'. Horrendous and atrocious must have flitted through his mind but been rejected!

Use of the voice

A lecture is not a formal oration nor is it a casual conversation; ideally, try to pitch the tone somewhere between the two. The voice should be warm and friendly, inviting the listener in rather than keeping him or her at a distance. Stave off monotony by making a conscious effort to introduce light and shade into your voice. The quickest way to bore your audience and lose their interest is by speaking in a monotone. Lift your voice at the beginning of a sentence and keep the tone upbeat; if you sound interested in what you are saying then the audience will respond and concentrate on your argument.

It's a good idea to be bold when addressing a group of people, even if you feel nervous inside. Stand tall, hold your head up high and speak out confidently and with purpose. Your voice will then sound energised and confident. Avoid undue emphasis: stress the words that need to be pointed up but don't come down heavily on every single word. It sounds incredibly tedious and does not make for easy listen. Overemphasis quickly leads to a hectoring tone and you don't want to fall into the trap of haranguing your audience.

Never underestimate the power of the pause! It gives the listeners a chance to digest what you have just said and provides you with a little breathing space before moving on to your next sentence or paragraph. It also enables you to be measured in style, appearing calm and confident and fully in control of yourself and your material. Think of yourself as a stately galleon rather than a speedboat!

I've spoken about the importance of lifting your voice when you are starting a new sentence or introducing a new thought. It is equally important to avoid dropping your voice at the end of a sentence, allowing the words to be lost in an unintelligible mumble. Once a listener has lost track of your meaning, interest and attention will soon waver.

Pronunciation

At the BBC we set great store by using the correct pronunciation for for-eign names and place names. The Pronunciation Unit enjoys a wonderful reputation in this field. It's worth remembering that it is a courtesy to pro-nounce someone's name correctly, so make an effort to find out the right pronunciation if you are including someone's name in your talk.

Avoid Americanisms if you can as they seem to arouse much ire in most British audiences! My particular *bete noire* is skedule rather than schedule. Also try to avoid eccentric or bizarre pronunciations as the listener tends to focus on them to the detriment of anything else you might be saying. I remember attending a lecture about D. H. Lawrence and becoming transfixed by the way the lecturer pronounced bosom as bazoom, with the stress on the second syllable, and novel as nuvvel. Consequently, I didn't learn a great deal about the complexities of *Sons and Lovers*!

Use of notes

We have a saying at Radio 4 that stands all announcers in good stead: 'en-gage brain before opening mouth'. To this end we tend to write a lot down, particularly when doing continuity work, in case a momentary brainstorm banishes the name of a well-known presenter from your mind just as you are introducing his or her programme, leaving you up the proverbial creek without a paddle. Having said that, however, do not fall into the trap of reciting your notes verbatim. Your words will lack spontaneity and may well fail to clarify your subject, let alone arouse interest. Notes in the form of a list of brief headings or key words will provide a useful springboard for your thoughts. A word of warning – make sure your notes are firmly secured in case Sod's Law sees to it that they are scattered to the four winds as you turn a page – I speak as a victim!

Controlling nerves

You will almost certainly give a better performance if you have a few nerves before delivering your lecture. They keep you on your mettle and prevent you from sounding bored and world-weary. The trick is to control them so that they work to your advantage, rather than allowing them to hamper your performance.

Always arrive early and allow yourself a few minutes of quiet contemplation; ideally, you want to achieve a state of calm control. Don't allow anything or anyone to fluster you or upset your equilibrium. I go in search of the loo – never give a lecture with a full bladder! – and run through some exercises. If you are feeling physically stressed give your arms a vigorous shake in the manner of Olympic swimmers. Bend over and let your body go floppy like a rag doll. In order to calm your breathing take a few slow, deep breaths and tell yourself as you breathe out 'I am calm' or 'I am in control'. Make a conscious effort to drop your shoulders. I find it useful to shut my eyes and count down very slowly from ten to one, imagining myself becoming lighter and floppier as I proceed. Sometimes I imagine colours as I count, moving from red through amber to green, by which time I hope to be ready for action! Just before you begin your lecture think of something funny that makes you laugh; this will relax you and make you smile inwardly. One other slightly frivolous word of advice – if your audience seem a little daunting as you stand before them, imagine them all naked. Nudity is a great leveller!

Summary

- Capture the interest and curiosity of your audience.
- Aim for brevity and clarity.
- Introduce light and shade into your voice and sound lively and enthusiastic.
- Take time before the talk to relax physically and mentally.

Chapter 10 **How to deal with questions**

Sir Alexander Macara

'We are in danger to be called in question'

Acts of the Apostles, xix, 40

It is to be hoped that readers will find that questions provide opportunities rather than dangers.

Like ancient Gaul, this chapter falls into three parts: how to answer questions after giving a presentation at a meeting; how to handle interviews from the 'media' and how to cope with a 'brains trust' or panel discussion.

Questions following a presentation

The story is told of an eminent physicist who had reluctantly accepted an invitation to address a predictably tiresome meeting. He was driven there by his favourite postgraduate student. On arrival, his disinclination to speak overcame any sense of obligation, and he decided to rest in his car while sending the student, armed with his PowerPoint presentation, to give the lecture. The eager acolyte coped competently with the presentation itself and with agreeably animated discussion until he was fazed by a particularly difficult challenge. 'The question is of rather too general a nature to require my expertise', he replied, 'but I will invite my chauffeur to deal with it.'

The credibility of the story aside, it does raise some salutary points. Obviously, one should try to avoid accepting unwelcome invitations and, if one has to delegate the invitation to a colleague, albeit armed with your prepared script, bear in mind that he might have problems dealing with questions. Moreover, care must be taken not to underestimate the intelligence or knowledge of the audience; invariably someone will know more about some aspects of the subject than the speaker.

How to Present at Meetings, Third Edition. Edited by George M. Hall and Neville Robinson.
© 2012 George M. Hall and Neville Robinson. Published 2012 by John Wiley & Sons, Ltd.

So, to our task. How should one approach audience's questions after a presentation?

- Prepare as for the presentation itself by seeking to master the subject. You can choose what to say or not to say in the presentation, but you can only speculate about questions, and 'being called in question' clearly presents more dangers than the presentation itself. Invited to address French professors of social medicine in the elegant Chateau de Longchamps in Paris about a European Association to which I wanted to recruit them, I was unexpectedly bidden to speak in French. All went well enough until questions came – more fast than thick. The chairman came to the rescue: 'They all speak English, mon ami, so it is only fair now to switch to your language.' The problem is, however, more often with the question itself than with the language in which it is couched, so one's preparation should not only cover the immediate ground of the subject but survey the hinterland. For example, if addressing 'clinical advances in late onset diabetes', one should review the epidemiology, the history of the diagnosis, treatment and management of the disease, together with its effect on the person as a whole, its relationship to other conditions, and its social, occupational and economic implications.
- Conduct a reconnaissance of the expected audience before preparing.
- Speculate about questions. Rehearse what you might choose to say in reply.
- On the day, dress up rather than down. Beverley Baxter once observed that 'by your dress you show respect'. Turning up in a dinner jacket and finding everyone else in casual smart attire, the late Sir John Brotherston – then CMO Scotland – explained, 'I have just come from the office'. Conversely, failing to wear a dinner jacket to a 'black tie dinner' is not so easily explained away. A jacket and tie can always be removed if appropriate; indeed, it may be effective after a formal presentation to slip off one's jacket before knuckling down to questions.
- Ascertain whether reporters are to be present and, if so, whom they represent. At a typically sparsely attended AGM that I was waiting to address, it was agreed that those attending should constitute the executive committee *en bloc*. The scrupulous secretary insisted on listing the names, thereby identifying an unknown young person as being from the medical newspaper, *PULSE*.
- Make your mark with the chairman: if a woman, ascertain whether she wishes to be addressed traditionally as 'Madam Chairman' or, as in contemporary parlance, as an inanimate object with four legs. The chairman has the power to make or break the occasion – and the speaker. If in doubt about any of the arrangements, seek the chairman's advice.

- Seek to give an impression of modest self-confidence; be positive, not negative. Allow an element of self-deprecation. Irony is acceptable, sarcasm is not.
- Speak simply, with appropriate colloquial language but not slang. Practise conciseness and clarity as distinct from brevity and oversimplification. Fluency is admirable but a stammer, which can suddenly afflict anyone in a difficult situation, can be turned to good account. The distinguished and much loved paediatrician, Freddie Miller, who had a particularly engaging stammer, used to relieve his hearers of any embarrassment by claiming that it was an advantage – 'it gives one time to think'.
- Indulge in spontaneous humour if you have the gift. Guard against giving gratuitous offence by insensitivity about age, gender, religion or race.
- Above all, try to keep calm under stress, however provoked you may be. A soft answer can turn away wrath and, more importantly, does nothing to diminish one's authority. Try to obtain, and maintain, eye contact with the audience throughout. Heaven defend one from the high platform, the scattered remote audience, the dim lighting, except, infuriatingly, in front of one's own eyes. In such a situation – sadly increasingly common – one can only do one's best. Ignore the spoiler who is muttering disapprovingly and speak directly to the empathetic listener.
- When the question is put, listen to it but try also to assess why it is asked; body language will often give a clue. Does the questioner genuinely want information or is he or she trying to impress? Be sensitive to the effect of your answer on the audience as a whole, including any reporters. In any event, answer the question that is asked (you are not a politician).
- Correct any mistaken assumptions in the question.
- The chairman may summarise, or seek to clarify, the question; beware of any change in its meaning or purpose, in which case your reply will call for diplomacy.
- Do not launch into a second presentation; leave people wanting more. Allow room for a supplementary question.
- If you consider the question stupid, be courteous and explain the relevant facts as though it had been sensible.
- If the question is too profound, you may have to regret that lack of time (has anyone ordered breakfast?) precludes a reply in depth. If the question is very wide, lack of time similarly precludes a reply in breadth.
- If the questioner is disconcertingly knowledgeable, you may invite his or her own opinion/explanation/information.
- What if one does not know the answer to the question? The celebrated Scots dramatist, James Bridie, a 'chronic' medical student in those halcyon days when universities were relaxed about examinations, when asked the

external relations of the knee joint, replied, 'I do not know the external relations of the knee joint, but the external relations of the elbow joint are . . . .' Not a bad try, but better to be honest and admit that you do not know. Ask if someone else can help – perhaps the questioner?

- How should you handle the individual who interrupts your presentation? You may have been forewarned about the bearded chap in a red shirt and green tie, and are therefore prepared. The chairman may come to the rescue but only you can decide whether or not to give way. Do either with good grace. An effective ploy is to claim that you are coming to that particular point later, whether or not you have any such intention.

On being interviewed

Keith Joseph was a disconcertingly honest intellectual, best remembered for his reorganisation of the National Health Service (NHS) as Secretary of State in the Health Administration in the early 1970s. The story is told of his first television interview in the early days of that revealing medium, when he was a new junior minister. He answered every question unguardedly, and had the insight at the end to observe that the interview had been disastrous. 'Yes, Sir Keith,' replied his interviewer, 'I am afraid it was.' 'Then we must do it again.' 'But, Sir Keith, it was *live*.' 'That is why I want do it again.'

Today's politicians are trained to deal with interviews, especially on television. Keith Joseph's experience reminds us of the crucial importance of knowing whether the interview is being recorded or broadcast 'live' or whether there may be an opportunity to see or hear it in advance and to make changes. As with questions from any audience, one needs to know who one's readers, listeners or viewers are likely to be, whom the interviewer is representing and what the objective of the interview is. It is wise to assume that interviewers are knowledgeable and that they may be hoping to present a preconceived angle. One also needs to know whether any colleagues – or others, especially if potential adversaries – are to be appearing alongside you and, if so, what contribution they are likely to make and what is to be the order of appearance. Prepare a number of points – five at most. However you may be provoked, try to remain studiously courteous, but cautious: exceptions prove the rule. Remember that it is *your* subject (or you should not be there) and *your* interview. The honour of your specialty, your practice, hospital or university, may be in your hands.

Your *aide memoire* should include the following additional points:

- Make your remarks appropriate to the audience, whether professional or general. Avoid jargon except for a specially knowledgeable audience.

- Correct any mistakes by the interviewer unless the matter is trivial and correction would be petty.
- Beware of pitfalls, for example, 'So what you are saying is ...' when it is not, or the multiple point question that is unanswerable in limited time; reply, 'The main point(s) is (are) ....'
- Take care with statistics: they should be told only when they are telling and if in doubt, leave them out. Keep them simple, for example 'half' rather than 'approximately 50 % give or take a point or two'.
- Do not say, 'I have x points' (although you do). You will look foolish when you fall short of the expected number.
- Never denigrate a rival or opponent.

The newspaper or journal interview
There are two specific related points:
1 Avoid talking 'off the record' or 'unattributably' even when invited to do so, unless you are very confident that the reporter is someone you can trust to resist the temptation to pull off a scoop on the strength of your indiscretion.
2 Assume that anything you say may be quoted.

The radio or television interview
Whichever the medium, try to ascertain how much time you will have. The duration of the interview may depend upon how cogent and convincing you are in reply to the first question. Television can be particularly brutal in cutting you off in mid-sentence either on the spot or in the cutting room. You may have to persuade the interviewer that you have something to say in order to secure the interview at all. The onus may be on you to secure a favourable interview. When Fergus Walsh, the veteran television interviewer, was reporting the profession's Core Values Conference in 1994, he was clearly sceptical as to whether we had anything 'new' to say. One was able to represent that, for the first time, the medical profession had explicitly acknowledged its responsibility, not only to individual patients and to the honour of the profession but to society as a whole, which led to the desired discussion about scarcity of resources and rationing.

There are rules, or at least tips, that are particularly relevant to radio and television:
- Say less rather than more; an arresting short reply to the opening question will invite further questions and secure more time to get your points across within the pre-set limit.

- Be prepared to back up your assertions or claims crisply with evidence or examples. Taking refuge in reassertion or waffle will leave you sounding or looking very foolish.
- Do not say, 'Speaking personally, I myself think ....' Tautology apart, 'I think' suggests you do not know. Do not start with 'well', or use fillers such as 'um. . ., er. . ., em. . .'. Avoid 'you know' like the plague – they do not, you are supposed to be telling them.
- Sound (and, on television, look) convincing and enthusiastic.
- Be pleasant to the interviewer whatever your true feelings. He (or she) can make you sound better or worse than you deserve.
- When you have finished, stop.

Each medium has its advantages and disadvantages. Hence, general rules apply to both, but there are specific points to bear in mind for each. Radio is less subject to distraction – for everyone concerned – than television. Radio puts a premium on the voice and television on the image. Vision can either distract from the message or enhance it. One's style of dress and address reinforce each other. Competent professionalism is the passport to success. Ignore the camera and look at the interviewer, who is usually more interesting; moreover, you need to read his or her body language. Do not fall for the pregnant pause and feel you have to fill a gap with some ill-considered irrelevance. Take care with your physical presentation. Stand erect with feet firmly on the ground or sit upright in your chair, not rocking it or yourself. Acknowledge your introduction and dismissal with a smile. You may be shown going about your business to set the scene for the interview. Appear brisk and business-like. It helps to carry an impressive-looking folder, but not a pile of books, which suggests that you cannot cope without a mobile library. Avoid steps.

The brains trust or panel

The eminent philosopher Professor Joad, a resident member of the original pre-television era BBC Brains Trust, once famously recast the question 'What is life?' as 'What *is* life?' The point of this anecdote is that a panel discussion is a different genre from the one-to-one question and answer session or interview. It often offers the opportunity to turn a question round in such a way as to give a more stimulating and useful answer than the original question permits. However, your answer should be no less relevant to the original question and should not be calculated to score over the other members of the panel, although it may have that effect. No matter, there is an inevitable element of rivalry – not always friendly – between the members of a panel, all of whom are anxious to reveal their knowledge or conceal their ignorance. 'The question is, which is to be master?' to quote Humpty Dumpty.

The challenge is to strike the right note. It is death to discussion for everyone to sing in unison, but discordant clashes can be equally destructive. Panel members should resist the temptation to interrupt their colleagues, however provoked, but should be prepared to respond when invited to help them out. Wit or originality always enhances proceedings, as does a telling anecdote. As in other situations, the chairman, however self-effacing, is the key figure, particularly in controlling anyone seeking to dominate proceedings and in encouraging less assertive participants. The chairman will usually decide upon the order of batting and move quickly to another member of the panel when one is stumped.

Sometimes the chairman will throw the question open and an instant decision is required. Do you jump in or wait? If you know the answer, have a go while the others are thinking; they will have to follow your lead or justify doing otherwise. If you do not have anything to say, save your breath in the hope that others will give you a clue or an opportunity to agree with them – the sincerest form of flattery – adding that you have nothing to add, which will please everyone, including the person waiting with contrived patience to pose the next question.

Let the last word be with Sir Toby Belch: 'I can say little more than I have studied.'

Summary

- When preparing a presentation, prepare for types of questions that might be asked afterwards.
- Make sure you cater for the particular audience you are addressing.
- When being interviewed prepare up to five points and try to remain courteous but cautious.
- If you are a member of a panel respond with a relevant answer and do not interrupt your colleagues.

Further reading

Media Tips. *BMA Public Affairs Division*, 2000.

Chapter 11 How not to give a presentation

Richard Smith

The invitation arrives. You are invited to speak on the same programme as the Pope, Bill Clinton, Madonna and Noam Chomsky. Beside yourself with excitement, you forget that you've had these sorts of invitations before and that for some strange reason none of the famous people ever turn up. They are all replaced by people you've never heard of who turn out to be even more boring than you. Having accepted the invitation, you get your own back by forgetting it completely. Two years later – 15 minutes before you are due to start speaking in Florence – you receive a phone call at your office in London asking where you are.

'I'm sorry,' you answer lamely, 'I forgot.'

'Don't worry,' answers the cheery voice at the end, 'We'll just ask Madonna to speak for 20 minutes longer. The audience of millionaire surgeons will be disappointed you're not here, but extra Madonna will be some compensation.'

Far from ruining this presentation, you may have improved the surgeons' conference, but forgetting altogether that you agreed to speak is a good way to make a mess of your presentation. A variant is to arrive late. Don't arrive too late because they will simply have cancelled your session, probably sending a thrill of pleasure through an audience facing the prospect of five consecutive speakers. The best thing is to arrive about 8 minutes late when the chairman has exhausted his puny supply of jokes and is just starting to introduce the next speaker. Rush up to the podium, waving your hands furiously and apologise profusely. If you can, trip over on the way. Once at the podium you can either spend 5 minutes searching for your notes or else say: 'I'm sorry, I've not had time to give my 87 slides to the man in the projector room.' Conversely, you could try saying, 'I'm sure that my PowerPoint presentation is on this disk somewhere,' as you project on to the screen a list of hundreds of similar file names.

How to Present at Meetings, Third Edition. Edited by George M. Hall and Neville Robinson.
© 2012 George M. Hall and Neville Robinson. Published 2012 by John Wiley & Sons, Ltd.

My initial point is that there are many, perhaps infinite, ways to give a bad presentation. Tolstoy writes in the first line of Anna Karenina that 'All happy families resemble one another, but each unhappy family is unhappy in its own way.' The same may be true for presentations. Good ones resemble each other, but bad ones come in many forms.

Preparing for a bad presentation

One way to prepare for a bad presentation is not to prepare at all. Step up to the plate, open your mouth, and see what comes out. With luck your talk will be an incoherent ramble. This is, however, a high-risk strategy because spontaneity may catch you out. Most medical presentations are so premeditated that spontaneity may inspire both your audience and you. Inspiration must be avoided at all costs. Similarly, you might be caught out by truth. 'I've been asked to promote this new drug but actually I'd be fearful of throwing it into the Thames because it might poison the few homunculus fish that survive there.' Truth is compelling to an audience, even if mumbled.

A really bad presentation needs careful preparation. A useful standby is to prepare for the wrong audience. If asked to speak to Italians, speak in German. If the audience is made up of 15-year-olds then prepare a complex talk that would baffle a collection of Nobel Prize winners. It's much the best strategy to give an overcomplicated presentation. 'Nobody ever lost money underestimating the public's intelligence,' said Barnum, Richard Nixon or somebody, and so you may be surprised by how well your grossly oversimplified presentation is received by your audience of professors.

Be sure to prepare a presentation that is the wrong length. Too long is much the best. Most of the audience will be delighted if your talk is too short, not least because it may provide more opportunity for them to hear their own voices. However, something that is too long always works, even if what you are saying is full of wit and wisdom.

Another trick is to ignore the topic you are given. Simply give the bad presentation that you have honed to the point of perfection by giving it time and time again and deleting anything that raises a flicker of interest. With luck most of the audience will have heard it several times before.

Extra help for your bad presentation is to send the organisers in advance a very long and dull CV. Your bad presentation may be given a tremendous boost by the chairman reading out your whole boring life story in a monotone. With luck you might find yourself beginning your presentation after you were supposed to finish. That always depresses an audience.

Aids to a bad presentation

When it comes to aids, standards are rising for those who want to give bad presentations. Indeed, it is probably impossible to give a truly awful presentation without aids. This is an area where new technology is enormously beneficial. First-rate bad presentations are usually multimedia: poorly filmed videos that are long and incomprehensible, tapes that are inaudible, music that is out of tune, props that can't be found and then break, and PowerPoint presentations that use every feature the software offers. Satellite links that keep breaking up can often be the icing on the cake of a bad presentation.

It's essential in the second decade of the new millennium to connect to the Internet during your bad presentation. You won't, of course, know the password for connecting and nor will anybody else in the room. While some willing soul goes to find somebody who does know the password simply look at your feet. When the person with the password arrives make sure that you have to go through dozens of highly complex screenshots to find the right one. In advance, make sure that your website isn't actually working. When everything freezes, say: 'Well, perhaps it wasn't that important anyway. I'll email you all the URL My full talk will be on the site, together with a video and a podcast.' The fact that your awful presentation will have an afterlife will strike dread into the audience.

Bad slides have long been the traditional standby of a bad presentation, but PowerPoint offers so many more possibilities. Preparing slides required premeditation and was costly. With PowerPoint you can be preparing dreadful slides up until the very moment when you open your mouth. The essence of a bad presentation in the old days was to have far too many slides and PowerPoint has made excess so much easier and cheaper. Indeed, PowerPoint has raised dramatically the standards of bad presentations. Speakers who once used a few, well-composed slides and spoke to the point have been seduced into prolixity and tedium by PowerPoint. Consequently it's become harder to be the worst speaker at a meeting.

Not only must you have far too many slides but also they must contain too much information and be too small for even those in the front row to read. Flash them up as fast as you can manage, making sure that they are in the wrong order with some upside down. Include lots of data and complicated graphs, and be sure to say at some point: 'I know that this slide breaks all the rules but . . . .' Ideally there should be little connection between what you are saying and what is on the slide. A good trick, especially with a politically correct audience, is to insert a slide of a naked woman and say something like 'My beautiful assistant is, I'm sure you will all agree, a little top heavy.' Don't, however, start a riot – otherwise your presentation will be universally agreed to be most memorable.

With PowerPoint be sure to use a wider range of fonts and colours and include moving and flashing signals to add to the complexity and subtract any meaning that might be getting through.

Unusual aids – such as animals or children – sometimes work. Try introducing all your children plus your pets and parents to the audience. Well done, it might make everybody cringe and create new highs in bad presentations.

Making your bad presentation

The essence of a bad presentation is to be boring. Anything that isn't boring will detract from your bad presentation. Don't wear interesting or unusual clothes. Never look at the audience. Mumble your presentation and preferably read it. A presentation that is read will usually be satisfyingly bad, but for the full effect you should have long complicated sentences with dozens of subclauses. Try for something as complex as Proust, but get the grammar wrong. Then put all the emphases in the wrong place to ensure that your audience can't understand what you're saying.

Try to torture your audience. Speak for about 10 minutes and then say: 'This is what I'm going to talk about.' Then after another 20 minutes say: 'I'm now coming to my central point. . ..' Ten minutes later, start saying 'Finally'. Say it at least five times in the next 15 minutes.

One of the best ways to be boring is to speak for too long. If the chairman tries to stop you, say something like 'This is very important.' You will, of course, make sure that it isn't important because important things may not be sufficiently boring. It's best to concentrate on the unimportant but to speak with great pomposity. Arrogance and pomposity always enhance a bad presentation. You could also try insulting your audience, but this could be dangerous – because it may become interesting. An electric atmosphere, even if it's electric with anger and embarrassment, is a sure sign that your bad presentation has failed.

Winding down

A truly bad presentation rarely produces any questions. Most people just want to get away. If you do get questions, you may have failed. However, all is not lost. By sticking to the basic rules of being boring and overcomplicated and speaking for too long you may be able to rescue your bad presentation. The extra rule on answering questions is that under no circumstances should you answer them. Once you have finished say: 'Does that answer your question?'

If the questioner has the affrontery to say 'no', then don't answer his question again – only at greater length. This formula can be repeated if necessary, but a third nonanswer is hardly ever needed.

This guide is written, you will have judged, from long experience. I've made all these mistakes – and more. Kurt Vonnegut boasts that he gave such bad lectures when a lecturer at New York University that he fell asleep during his own lectures. I remember giving a lecture in Manchester on creativity in science where the entire audience was almost unconscious and I suddenly thought: 'This is rubbish, utter rubbish.' I was tempted to stop and say: 'You're not enjoying this and nor am I. Let's stop and go down the pub.' I didn't and thank goodness that I didn't – otherwise it wouldn't have been an outstandingly bad presentation.

Summary

- Good presentations resemble each other but bad ones come in many forms.
- Lack of preparation, preparation for the wrong audience, making the talk too long and ignoring the topic all contribute to a bad presentation.
- Visual aids of poor quality, which are too numerous or with too much information, are almost *de rigeur* for a poor presentation.
- Mumbling, reading from a script and lack of eye contact will all help.
- A bad presentation rarely produces any questions, but if it does be sure not to answer them directly.

Chapter 12 **How to chair a session**

Roger Horton

Chairing a session at a scientific meeting is like so many things in life – do a good job and no one will notice you or remember your name, but do a bad job and you will be blamed for everything, including the incoherent speaker who left his slides at home. The key to successfully chairing a session is to do your homework thoroughly.

What type of meeting?

The role and responsibilities of the chairman will be coloured by the type of meeting. Often you begin to learn the trade at a small, one-day learned society meeting by chairing a short session of free communications, delivered by junior colleagues. The venue is probably familiar, the audience small, the atmosphere supportive and the speakers petrified! A natural progression is to the larger, national conference, spread over several days with parallel sessions, and with a more intense and sometimes adversarial atmosphere.

In attempting to offer advice, I have selected what many would consider the 'worst case scenario'. The meeting is a large prestigious world congress, held overseas. You have agreed to chair a half-day symposium, comprising six speakers, in an area with which you are familiar, but not an expert. The venue is a conference centre, also using several local hotels, in a city not known to you. You did not organise the symposium and none of the speakers is known to you. International reputations, including yours, may be built and lost in such situations. In dealing with this (unlikely) set of circumstances I will set out the principles and timing that the reader can adapt to less demanding situations.

How to Present at Meetings, Third Edition. Edited by George M. Hall and Neville Robinson.
© 2012 George M. Hall and Neville Robinson. Published 2012 by John Wiley & Sons, Ltd.

First principle: get started early

Three months before the meeting

Get to know your speakers and their work. The mechanics are simple these days. As a starting point, search by name one of the many bibliographic databases. Print off a list of publications, identify those related to the subject of the meeting and read them. This should help you establish the standing of the speakers, how long they have worked in this particular field, areas of controversy and recent advances.

Two months before the meeting

By now the meeting abstracts will be printed and the organisers may well have sent you, as chairman, copies of the abstracts of the speakers in your session. If not, request them, together with mail, telephone and e-mail contacts for the speakers.

Make contact with the speakers, preferably by e-mail. Send contact details and copies of abstracts to all speakers and encourage them to make contact with each other, even to exchange slides (one advantage of PowerPoint is the ability to send slides around the world as e-mail attachments – some people argue it's the only advantage). The purpose of all this electronic interchange is to ensure a coherent programme and to prevent each speaker giving essentially the same introduction. In the event of a disagreement, you are the referee.

With computer-generated slides universally used for presentations, it is important to find out from the organisers:

- What formats will be supported (PC, Mac)?
- What presentation packages (Microsoft PowerPoint only or others) will be supported and what versions?
- What media will be supported? USB flash drives (or memory sticks as they are commonly referred to) are almost universally the preferred media these days, but CD and DVD are still used.
- Will speakers be able to use their own laptops? This may be important if presentations include video clips. Mac users (an underpriveledged class) tend to be slightly paranoid and always prefer their own laptops.

Although there are fewer problems with compatibility these days, they do still happen and I think it is worth encouraging the speakers to bring their laptops, complete with software packages and presentations; if things do go wrong, they can always download the slides again.

At this stage you need to ensure that all participants are absolutely clear about the venue and date and time of the symposium and, above all, the duration of their contribution (for example, 25 minutes allowed to speak and 10 minutes for questions). Ask speakers to arrive 15 minutes before the start of the session for a briefing. It is also good at this point to ask contributors for copies of papers in press. This avoids any surprises at a later date.

If circumstances allow, I try to organise a social event for the speakers on the day before the session. This may be just meeting for coffee in the conference centre or going out for a meal. This is particularly valued by junior speakers who can be overawed by speaking on the same programme as 'superstars'. It is helpful to get agreement for this before the meeting. The local organisers will usually suggest appropriate venues and may even make bookings.

One to two days before the session
Venue-related
Make an effort to attend other sessions in the same venue. It is important that you, as chairman, are clear about the technical aspects of the arrangements and are able to inform the speakers authoritatively. It also gives you an opportunity to learn from other people's mistakes.

What should I be looking for?
- Are microphones necessary for speakers? Are they podium-mounted or attached to the speaker?
- Can speakers be clearly heard? Sit in different parts of the auditorium to find out.
- Do the technicians have a good command of the English language.
- Do the arrangements for slides work well? They have to, because there is nothing more disastrous for a meeting than major foul-ups with slides.
- Do members of the audience need to use microphones when asking questions? Are there sufficient numbers? Are they easily identified?
- Can the platform and the audience hear the questions?
- Is the venue easy to find and well signposted?
- Is there a technician present throughout? If not, how can one be contacted in an emergency?
- Is the room a comfortable temperature and adequately ventilated?

Some might regard the above as unnecessary, over-fussy and not the responsibility of the chairman. However, it is clear that if you are able to identify potential problems in advance you have a chance of fixing them; if you find out on the day, you have no chance.

Speaker-related
One of the greatest anxieties of chairing a meeting, particularly if you are also an organiser, is: Will the speakers actually show up?

Checking with the meeting secretariat that the speakers have registered (and therefore arrived) can help to allay these fears. At the same time, you can obtain details of their local accommodation to confirm the time and venue of any social function and of the meeting.

Remind speakers to arrive 15 minutes before the session is due to start for a briefing.

On the day

- Arrive at least half an hour before the session is due to start.
- Make sure any notices are displayed.
- Make yourself known to the technician and ensure slides have been handed in from all speakers (it is now usual for this to be done the day before for morning sessions or early morning for afternoon sessions). Check that each presentation is clearly identified. Ensure that slides have been checked. Ensure that the technician knows the running order.
- Check that any special requirements are in place.
- Check the sound and the laser pointer (have a spare laser pointer about your person).
- Check that there is an adequate supply of water and clean glasses.
- It can be helpful to the audience to display a slide with the title of the session. How many times have you found yourself sitting in the wrong room?
- Hold a briefing session for speakers 15 minutes before the session is due to start. This should include: introductions for any participants who have not previously met; making technical arrangements for slides, sound and lights; reiterating the timing and advising speakers on how you will indicate when they have 5 minutes left and when their time is up (visual cues are often the best); having a reassuring word with the junior and less-experienced speakers; and attending to bodily functions – you may be in the room for 2 hours.

So at last you are all set to go.

- Start the session on time. If you are unable to keep to time, don't expect your speakers to do so.
- Introduce yourself and any co-chairman, welcome the audience and out-line any housekeeping details (coffee breaks, meals, etc.). Sometimes the chairman gives a brief introduction to the session. Make it brief.
- Introduce the presentations by title and by speaker.
- Ensure that the speakers stick to time. An overrun of 1 minute into a 5-minute discussion session or 3 minutes into a 10-minute discussion session is the maximum that should be allowed. If speakers ignore your visual cues, you must interrupt, politely but firmly, requesting the speakers to conclude their presentations. It is very unprofessional and discourteous for speakers to overrun. They are effectively saying that what I have to say is more important than what the other speakers have to say. It is your job to

prevent this. At the end of each presentation, thank the speaker and request questions or comments. Identify those wishing to ask questions and request that they identify themselves and their affiliation. Ensure that the audience are able to hear the question and repeat the question if necessary:

- Encourage brief questions – do not allow the questioner to give a lecture.
- Encourage brief answers – do not allow the speaker to give another lecture.
- Try to ensure that all questioners get an opportunity (time permitting). If time runs out, make a mental note of who was unable to ask their questions and try to give them an opportunity to ask questions later.
- Ensure that one or two individuals do not hog the questioning.
- If the discussion gets too heated, then it is your job to cool it down with a diplomatic intervention.
- Ensure that you always have one or two questions ready should the audience be stunned into silence. This is unusual but it does happen, and a little forward planning prevents embarrassment for the speaker and the chairman.
- Keep to time. Curtailment of coffee and lunch breaks to catch up is invariably unpopular with catering staff and the audience.

At the end of the session

- Publicly thank speakers, organisers, sponsors and audience. A private word of thanks to each of the speakers and to technical staff is usually greatly appreciated.
- Congratulate yourself on a job well done (no one else will) and enjoy the rest of the meeting.

Summary

- The key to successfully chairing a session is to do your homework thoroughly.
- The role and responsibilities of the chair will be coloured by the type of meeting.
- Get to know your speakers and their work a few months before the meeting.
- Identify what visual aids the speakers will be using and familiarise yourself with the technical arrangements of the venue.
- On the day of the session, get there early to check that everything is organised and running to schedule.
- Ensure that the speakers keep to their allotted time.

Index

How to Present at Meetings, Third Edition. Edited by George M. Hall and Neville Robinson.
© 2012 George M. Hall and Neville Robinson. Published 2012 by John Wiley & Sons, Ltd.